THE UNTOLD TRUTH ABOUT HEART DISEASE

A Comprehensive Guide to Understanding and Preventing Cardiovascular Issues

BROOKLYN LUCAS

All rights reserved. No part of this book may be copied, shared, or transmitted in any way, whether by photocopying, recording, or other electronic or mechanical means, without the publisher's prior written consent. This excludes brief quotations used in critical reviews and certain other noncommercial uses allowed by copyright law.

This book is designed for educational and informational purposes only. The content aims to enhance understanding and appreciation of health-related topics. Any references to specific events, names, or copyrighted materials are included for commentary, criticism, or review.

The author and publisher are not responsible for any negative effects that may arise, directly or indirectly, from the information provided in this book.

TABLE OF CONTENT

INTRODUCTION

The human heart. A fist-sized marvel that tirelessly pumps lifeblood throughout our bodies, a silent conductor orchestrating the symphony of our existence. Yet, its strength can be surprisingly fragile, and its rhythm disrupted by a multitude of unseen forces. This book is not just about understanding those forces, the silent threats that lurk beneath the surface, but about empowering you to become the custodian of your own heart's well-being.

My journey into the world of heart health wasn't a textbook case. It wasn't fueled by abstract statistics or distant research papers. It was ignited by the very real fear gripping me as I watched my friend, Tina, battle a silent enemy within her own chest.

Tina– vibrant, witty, with a laugh that could fill a room – wasn't someone you'd associate with heart disease. She was active, health-conscious, a picture of youthful vitality. But then came the day when a seemingly ordinary walk in the park turned into a terrifying ordeal. Crushing chest pain, a cold sweat, and a gnawing fear that clawed its way into her eyes. The hospital confirmed the unthinkable – a coronary artery blockage, a ticking time bomb waiting to explode.

The following weeks were a blur of tests, consultations, and a rollercoaster of emotions. Witnessing Tina grapple with her diagnosis, the fear etched on her face, the uncertainty clouding her future, was a turning point for me. It was a stark reminder that heart disease doesn't discriminate. It can strike anyone, at any time.

But Tina's story isn't just about fear. It's also about resilience. The way she embraced the changes necessary to manage her condition, the unwavering support she received from loved ones, and the newfound determination that shone in her eyes – it all sparked a fire within me. I knew I had to sift deeper, to understand this silent threat, to equip myself and others with the knowledge to protect our most vital organ.

This book is the culmination of that journey. It's a comprehensive guide, a roadmap to navigating the complexities of heart health. We'll explore the "untold truths" about heart disease, debunk myths, and shed light on the often-overlooked factors that influence your heart's well-being.

More importantly, we'll empower you to take charge. You'll learn about preventative measures, discover strategies for managing existing conditions, and jump into the cutting-edge advancements shaping the future of heart care.

This isn't just a book or textbook; it's a call to action. It's a call to listen to the whispers of your heart, to understand its vulnerabilities, and to champion its well-being. Together, let's rewrite the narrative, ensure that heart disease doesn't steal the laughter, the joy, and the vibrant life that pulsates within us all.

CHAPTER ONE

THE MIGHTY ENGINE: UNDERSTANDING YOUR HEART

"The heart has its reasons which reason knows nothing of." - Blaise Pascal, French philosopher and mathematician.

This enigmatic quote by Pascal perfectly encapsulates the complex and fascinating nature of the human heart. Long revered as the seat of emotions and the very essence of life, the heart is far more than just a poetic symbol. It's a tirelessly working, intricate biological machine responsible for the very foundation of our existence.

Every single beat, estimated at a staggering 100,000 per day, propels life-giving blood throughout a vast network of vessels, nourishing every cell and organ in our bodies. But beneath this seemingly straightforward function lies a world of intricate mechanisms, electrical impulses, and a remarkable capacity for adaptation.

The Symphony of Life: Anatomy and Function

Imagine a muscular fist, roughly the size of your closed hand, nestled within the protective cage of your ribs. This is your heart, a marvel of engineering composed of four distinct chambers working in perfect harmony. The upper chambers, the atria, act as receiving chambers, collecting blood returning from the body. The lower chambers, the ventricles, are the powerhouses, their muscular walls contracting rhythmically to pump blood throughout the circulatory system.

But the heart doesn't operate in isolation. A complex network of valves ensures one-way blood flow, directing it through the correct chambers and preventing backflow. These valves, akin to tiny gates, open and close with each beat, their delicate dance maintaining the vital flow of life.

The magic, however, extends beyond mere muscle and valves. The heart conducts its own silent symphony, thanks to a specialized electrical conduction system. Specialized cells generate electrical impulses that travel across the heart's surface, triggering coordinated contractions of the atria and ventricles. This intricate electrical choreography ensures a smooth, rhythmic pumping action, vital for optimal blood circulation.

Beyond the Pump: The Heart's Untold Secrets

While the heart's role as a pump is undeniable, recent research has shed light on some of its "untold truths." We're now discovering the heart is an intelligent organ, capable of sensing and responding to various stimuli. It houses its own nervous system, influencing not just its own function but also other bodily systems.

The heart also plays a crucial role in the immune system, producing white blood cells essential for fighting off infections. Additionally, research suggests the heart may even contribute to emotional regulation, highlighting the profound mind-body connection.

The Untold Threats: Beyond Cholesterol

For decades, the focus of heart health has primarily revolved around cholesterol management. However, the landscape is changing. We're now realizing that heart disease is a complex interplay of various risk factors, some of them "untold" stories waiting to be addressed.

One such factor is chronic inflammation. Think of inflammation as a fire burning silently within your body. It can damage blood vessels, promote plaque buildup, and increase heart disease risk. Factors like chronic stress, unhealthy diet, and even gum disease can all contribute to this inflammatory state.

Another "untold truth" lies in the world within your gut. The gut microbiome, a vast ecosystem of trillions of bacteria, plays a crucial role in overall health, including heart health. Emerging research suggests an imbalanced gut microbiome may contribute to inflammation and other risk factors for heart disease.

Understanding these "untold truths" empowers us to take a more holistic approach to heart health. It's not just about monitoring cholesterol; it's about managing stress, maintaining a healthy gut, and addressing all the factors that can silently contribute to heart disease risk.

1.1 The Heart's Anatomy and Function

Forget the clunky gears and pistons of a car engine. The human heart is a marvel of biological engineering, a consonance of muscle, valves, and electrical impulses working in seamless coordination to sustain life. Imagine a muscular fist, roughly the size of your closed hand, nestled securely within the protective cage of your ribs. That's your heart, tirelessly pumping life-giving blood throughout a vast network of vessels, nourishing every cell and organ in your body. But beneath this seemingly straightforward function lies a world of intricate chambers, valves acting like silent guardians, and a remarkable electrical system that conducts the rhythm of life.

Let's dig deeper into this remarkable organ, dissecting its anatomy and understanding the magic behind each beat.

The Four Chambers: A Coordinated Dance

Think of your heart as a four-roomed house, each chamber playing a specific role in the blood circulation process. The upper two chambers, the atria (singular: atrium), are known as the receiving chambers. Picture them as entryways. Deoxygenated blood returning from your body via the superior and inferior vena cavae enters the right atrium. Meanwhile, oxygen-rich blood returning from your lungs flows into the left atrium through the pulmonary veins.

The real powerhouses lie below – the ventricles. These muscular chambers, particularly the left ventricle, are responsible for the forceful pumping action that propels blood throughout the body. Imagine them as the engines, fueled by oxygen-rich blood, ready to send it on its life-sustaining journey.

The Guardians of Flow: One-Way Valves

But how does blood ensure a smooth, one-way flow within this four-chambered house? Enter the valves, acting as silent guardians at the doorways between chambers and blood vessels. These intricate structures, composed of thin flaps of tissue, open and close with each heartbeat, meticulously directing blood flow.

The tricuspid valve, located between the right atrium and ventricle, ensures deoxygenated blood flows from the right atrium into the right ventricle. It's like a one-way door, preventing blood from backflowing into the atrium. Similarly, the mitral valve guards the passage between the left atrium and ventricle, ensuring oxygen-rich blood enters the powerful left ventricle.

Once the ventricles contract, a different set of valves comes into play. The pulmonic valve, positioned between the right ventricle and pulmonary artery, prevents blood from flowing back into the ventricle as it exits towards the lungs for oxygenation. Likewise, the aortic valve, located between the left ventricle and aorta, ensures the forceful ejection of oxygenated blood into the aorta, the body's main artery, for distribution to all organs and tissues.

The Electrical Conductor: Orchestrating the Rhythm

The heart doesn't operate in a haphazard manner. Each beat, each coordinated contraction of atria and ventricles, is orchestrated by a specialized electrical conduction system. Nestled within the right atrium lies a cluster of specialized cells called the sinoatrial node (SA node), also known as the heart's natural pacemaker. These cells act like a conductor, spontaneously generating electrical impulses.

These electrical impulses travel across a pathway in the right atrium, triggering the atria to contract simultaneously. The impulse then reaches another specialized group of cells, the atrioventricular node (AV node), located between the atria and ventricles. The AV node acts like a relay station, briefly delaying the signal before sending it down specialized pathways to the ventricles. This delay allows the atria to complete their contraction and fully empty blood into the ventricles before the powerful ventricles contract to pump blood out.

Finally, the electrical impulse spreads through a network of fibers within the ventricles, causing them to contract in a coordinated fashion. This coordinated contraction of atria and ventricles, orchestrated by the electrical conduction system, is what we feel as our heartbeat, the tireless rhythm of life.

Beyond the Pump: The Heart's Untold Complexities

The story of the heart, however, extends beyond its role as a mere pump. Recent research has revealed some fascinating "untold truths" about this remarkable organ. We're now discovering that the heart is an intelligent organ, capable of sensing and responding to various stimuli. It houses its own nervous system, influencing not just its own function but also other bodily systems.

For instance, the heart can detect changes in blood pressure and adjust its pumping rate accordingly. It can also sense hormones like adrenaline released during stress and respond by increasing heart rate and contractility to meet the body's increased demands. This intricate communication between the heart and other systems highlights the profound mind-body connection.

The heart also plays a crucial role in the immune system, producing white blood cells essential for fighting off infections. Additionally, research suggests the heart may even contribute to emotional regulation. Studies have shown that positive emotions can have a beneficial effect on heart rate variability, a measure of the heart's ability to adapt to changing conditions.

1.2 The Electrical Orchestration: Heart Rhythm and Conduction

Forget the clunky gears and pistons of a car engine. The human heart is an orchestra of life, a symphony of muscle, valves, and electrical impulses working in seamless coordination to sustain existence. Imagine a muscular fist, roughly the size of your closed hand, nestled securely within the protective cage of your ribs. That's your heart, tirelessly pumping life-giving blood throughout a vast network of vessels, nourishing every cell and organ in your body. But beneath this seemingly straightforward function lies a world of intricate chambers, valves acting like silent guardians, and a remarkable electrical system that conducts the rhythm of life.

Let's explore this remarkable organ in greater depth, dissecting its anatomy and understanding the magic behind each beat.

The Four Chambers: A Coordinated Dance

Think of your heart as a four-roomed house, each chamber playing a specific role in the blood circulation process. The upper two chambers, the atria (singular: atrium), are known as the receiving chambers. Picture them as entryways. Deoxygenated blood returning from your body via the superior and inferior vena cavae enters the right atrium. Meanwhile, oxygen-rich blood returning from your lungs flows into the left atrium through the pulmonary veins. (See accompanying Figure 1)

[Figure 1: Labeled diagram of the human heart showing the four chambers, superior and inferior vena cavae, and pulmonary veins]

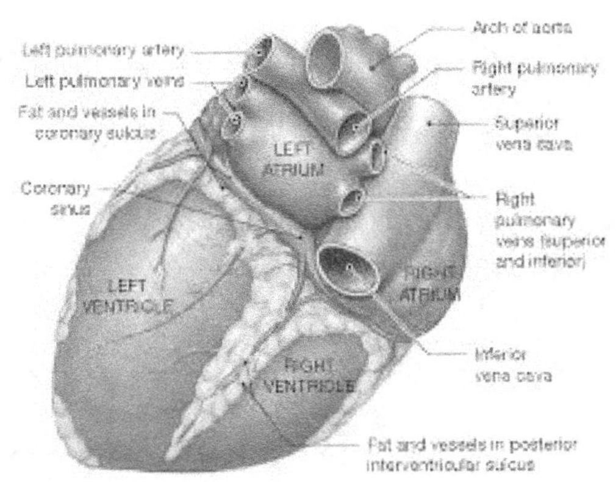

The real powerhouses lie below – the ventricles. These muscular chambers, particularly the left ventricle, are responsible for the forceful pumping action that propels blood throughout the body. Imagine them as the engines, fueled by oxygen-rich blood, ready to send it on its life-sustaining journey.

The Guardians of Flow: One-Way Valves

But how does blood ensure a smooth, one-way flow within this four-chambered house? Enter the valves, acting as silent guardians at the doorways between chambers and blood vessels. These intricate structures, composed of thin flaps of tissue, open and close with each heartbeat, meticulously directing blood flow.

The tricuspid valve, located between the right atrium and ventricle, ensures deoxygenated blood flows from the right atrium into the right ventricle. It's like a one-way door, preventing blood from backflowing into the atrium. Similarly, the mitral valve guards the passage between the left atrium and ventricle, ensuring oxygen-rich blood enters the powerful left ventricle.

Once the ventricles contract, a different set of valves comes into play. The pulmonic valve, positioned between the right ventricle and pulmonary artery, prevents blood from flowing back into the ventricle as it exits towards the lungs for oxygenation. Likewise, the aortic valve, located between the left ventricle and aorta, ensures the forceful ejection of oxygenated blood into the aorta, the body's main artery, for distribution to all organs and tissues.

The Electrical Conductor: Orchestrating the Rhythm

The heart doesn't operate in a haphazard manner. Each beat, each coordinated contraction of atria and ventricles, is orchestrated by a specialized electrical conduction system. Nestled within the right atrium lies a cluster of specialized cells called the sinoatrial node (SA node), also known as the heart's natural pacemaker. These cells act like a conductor, spontaneously generating electrical impulses.

These electrical impulses travel across a pathway in the right atrium, triggering the atria to contract simultaneously. The impulse then reaches another specialized group of cells, the atrioventricular node (AV node), located between the atria and ventricles. The AV node acts like a relay station, briefly delaying the signal before sending it down specialized pathways to the ventricles. This delay allows the atria to complete their contraction and fully empty blood into the ventricles before the powerful ventricles contract to pump blood out. (See accompanying Figure 2)

[Figure 2: Labeled diagram of the heart's electrical conduction system, including the SA node, AV node, and bundle of His]

Finally, the electrical impulse spreads through a network of fibers within the ventricles, causing them to contract in a coordinated fashion. This coordinated contraction of atria and ventricles, orchestrated by the electrical conduction system, is what we feel as our heartbeat, the tireless rhythm of life.

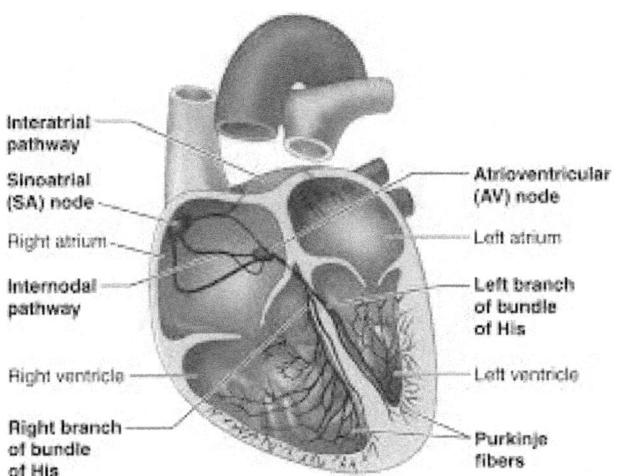

Interatrial pathway
Sinoatrial (SA) node
Right atrium
Internodal pathway
Right ventricle
Right branch of bundle of His
Atrioventricular (AV) node
Left atrium
Left branch of bundle of His
Left ventricle
Purkinje fibers

CHAPTER TWO

THE SILENT THREAT: RECOGNIZING DIFFERENT TYPES OF HEART DISEASE

"The greatest wealth is health." - Virgil, Roman poet.

This simple quote by Virgil holds immense truth, particularly when considering the irreplaceable role of the heart in our overall well-being. Heart disease, often referred to as cardiovascular disease (CVD), remains the leading cause of death globally, claiming millions of lives each year. But unlike a single, monolithic entity, heart disease encompasses a spectrum of conditions, each with its unique characteristics and potential consequences. Understanding these different types of heart disease empowers us to recognize the silent threats lurking beneath the surface and take proactive steps towards prevention and management.

Coronary Artery Disease: The Culprit Behind Heart Attacks

Coronary artery disease (CAD) is often the first condition that comes to mind when we think of heart disease. It arises from a gradual buildup of plaque, a fatty substance, within the coronary arteries. These arteries are responsible for supplying oxygen-rich blood to the heart muscle itself. As plaque accumulates, it narrows the arteries, restricting blood flow. This restricted blood flow can lead to angina, a condition characterized by chest pain or discomfort that occurs when the heart muscle doesn't receive enough oxygen. In its most severe form, a complete blockage of a coronary artery can trigger a heart attack, a life-threatening event where a portion of the heart muscle is deprived of oxygen and nutrients, leading to tissue death.

Beyond Blockages: A Broader Spectrum of Threats

While coronary artery disease is a major culprit, the story of heart disease doesn't end there. Let's explore some other conditions that fall under the umbrella of cardiovascular disease:

Heart Failure: This doesn't imply the heart has stopped functioning entirely. Instead, heart failure refers to a condition where the heart muscle is weakened or damaged, compromising its ability to pump blood effectively. This can lead to a buildup of fluid in the lungs and other tissues, causing shortness of breath, fatigue, and swelling.

Heart Valve Disease: The heart's valves, as we learned earlier, ensure a smooth, one-way flow of blood. However, these valves can malfunction due to various reasons, including infection, wear and tear, or a congenital defect present at birth. A malfunctioning valve can either narrow the opening (stenosis), restrict blood flow, or allow blood to leak backward (regurgitation). Both scenarios can place strain on the heart and lead to other complications.

Arrhythmias: The heart's rhythm is a meticulously orchestrated dance. Arrhythmias disrupt this rhythm, causing the heart to beat too slowly (bradycardia), too quickly (tachycardia), or irregularly. While some arrhythmias might be benign, others can be life-threatening, requiring immediate medical attention.

Cardiomyopathy: This term refers to a disease of the heart muscle itself, primarily affecting its structure and function. Different types of cardiomyopathies can weaken the heart muscle, impair its pumping efficiency, and lead to heart failure.

Congenital Heart Defects: Sometimes, the heart's structure may develop abnormally before birth. These congenital heart defects can range from mild to severe, affecting blood flow through the heart and requiring medical intervention or surgery.

The Silent Threat: Recognizing the Warning Signs

One of the most concerning aspects of heart disease is its ability to progress silently for years. Symptoms may not appear until the condition is already advanced. However, being aware of the potential warning signs can empower you to seek medical attention early on, potentially preventing complications.

Here are some general warning signs of heart disease to be mindful of:

- Chest pain, pressure, or tightness
- Shortness of breath, especially with exertion
- Palpitations, feeling like your heart is racing or fluttering
- Pain or discomfort radiating to the arm, jaw, shoulder, or back
- Lightheadedness, dizziness, or fainting
- Unusual fatigue or weakness
- Swelling in the ankles or feet

It's important to remember that these symptoms can also be caused by other conditions. However, if you experience any of them, particularly if they are persistent or worsening, don't hesitate to consult your doctor for a proper evaluation.

Early Detection is Key: The Power of Preventive Measures

The good news is that many forms of heart disease are preventable or manageable. By adopting a healthy lifestyle and addressing risk factors, you can significantly reduce your chances of developing heart disease or slow its progression. Here are some key strategies to consider:

- Maintain a healthy weight: Excess weight puts additional strain on your heart. Aim for a healthy weight through a balanced diet and regular physical activity.

- Embrace a heart-healthy diet: Focus on a diet rich in fruits, vegetables, whole grains, and lean protein. Limit saturated and trans fats, cholesterol, and added sodium.

- Get regular exercise: Aim for at least 150 minutes of moderate-intensity exercise or 75 minutes of vigorous-intensity exercise per week.

2.1 coronary artery disease (CAD): The Culprit Behind Heart Attacks

Coronary artery disease, with its infamous plaque buildup, is a major villain in the heart disease story. But the plot thickens when we delve deeper into the spectrum of cardiovascular conditions silently threatening our well-being. Let's study some lesser-known yet significant players in this drama.

Heart Failure: When the Engine Falters

Imagine your heart as a tireless pump, constantly pushing blood throughout your body. Now, picture that pump weakening, struggling to keep up with the demands placed upon it. This, in essence, is what happens in heart failure.

Heart failure doesn't imply the heart has stopped working entirely. Instead, it signifies a condition where the heart muscle is weakened or damaged, compromising its ability to pump blood effectively. This weakening can arise from various culprits:

- Coronary artery disease: As discussed earlier, CAD can damage the heart muscle by depriving it of oxygen-rich blood.

- High blood pressure: Uncontrolled high blood pressure forces the heart to work harder over time, eventually leading to weakening.

- Heart valve disease: Malfunctioning valves can place a strain on the heart muscle as it tries to overcome the resistance to blood flow.

- Cardiomyopathy: This condition directly affects the heart muscle itself, weakening its structure and function.

- Viral infections: Certain viruses can infect the heart muscle, causing inflammation and weakening.

The consequences of heart failure can be debilitating. As the heart struggles to pump efficiently, blood can back up in the circulatory system. This backup can lead to a buildup of fluid in the lungs (pulmonary edema) causing shortness of breath, particularly when lying down.

Additionally, fluid can accumulate in other tissues, leading to swelling in the ankles and feet.

Heart Failure: A Spectrum of Severity

Heart failure isn't a one-size-fits-all condition. It exists on a spectrum, ranging from mild to severe. In the early stages, symptoms may be subtle, like fatigue or shortness of breath during exertion. As the condition progresses, symptoms become more pronounced and can significantly impact daily activities.

However, the good news is that heart failure can often be managed effectively. Early diagnosis and treatment can significantly improve quality of life and prevent complications. Treatment strategies typically involve medication to manage symptoms, lifestyle modifications like diet and exercise, and sometimes medical procedures or surgery.

Heart Valve Disease: The Guardians Under Siege

Remember the valves in your heart, those silent guardians ensuring one-way blood flow? Unfortunately, these valves can malfunction due to various reasons, disrupting the smooth flow of blood.

Several culprits can contribute to heart valve disease:

Age-related wear and tear: As we age, the valves can become stiff or thickened, compromising their ability to open and close properly.

Rheumatic fever: This complication of a bacterial infection can damage the heart valves, particularly in children.

Congenital heart defects: Sometimes, babies are born with heart valves that don't develop normally.

There are two main ways a heart valve can malfunction:

- Stenosis: This occurs when the valve opening narrows, restricting blood flow. Depending on the severity, stenosis can cause symptoms like fatigue, shortness of breath, chest pain, or heart palpitations.
- Regurgitation: This happens when the valve doesn't close tightly, allowing blood to leak backward. This

leakage forces the heart to work harder to pump blood forward, leading to eventual weakening.

Heart valve disease, if left untreated, can have serious consequences. It can lead to heart failure, irregular heartbeats, and even heart attack. However, the good news is that various treatment options are available depending on the severity and type of valve dysfunction. These may include medication, minimally invasive procedures to repair the valve, or valve replacement surgery.

Arrhythmias: When the Rhythm Goes Rogue

Our hearts beat in a specific rhythm, a coordinated dance between the atria and ventricles. This rhythm is orchestrated by the electrical conduction system. However, sometimes, this system malfunctions, leading to arrhythmias, or irregular heartbeats.

Arrhythmias can manifest in various ways:

- Bradycardia: This refers to a heart rate that is too slow, typically below 60 beats per minute. While some athletes may have naturally slow heart rates without any problems, bradycardia can sometimes cause fatigue, dizziness, or fainting.

- Tachycardia: This signifies a heart rate that is too fast, exceeding 100 beats per minute at rest. Tachycardia can cause palpitations, chest pain, shortness of breath, and anxiety.

- Premature ventricular contractions (PVCs): These are extra heartbeats that originate in the ventricles, causing a fluttering sensation in the chest.

- Atrial fibrillation (AFib): This is a common type of arrhythmia where the upper chambers of the the upper chambers of the heart, the atria, beat irregularly and chaotically. This disrupts the normal flow of blood from the atria to the ventricles and can lead to blood clots forming in the stagnant blood within the atria. These clots, if dislodged, can travel through the bloodstream and lodge in vital organs like the brain, causing a stroke – a major complication of AFib. Additionally, AFib can weaken the heart's pumping efficiency and contribute to heart failure.

People with AFib may experience symptoms like heart palpitations, shortness of breath, fatigue, and lightheadedness. However, for some individuals, AFib may have no noticeable symptoms at all, making it crucial for regular checkups and screenings, especially for those at higher risk.

Cardiomyopathy: When the Heart Muscle Itself Weakens

- The term cardiomyopathy refers to a disease of the heart muscle itself. It affects the structure and function of the heart muscle, hindering its ability to pump blood effectively. There are several types of cardiomyopathies, each with its own cause and characteristics:

- Dilated cardiomyopathy: This is the most common type, causing the heart muscle to enlarge and weaken, compromising its pumping ability. The exact cause of dilated cardiomyopathy is often unknown, but it can be linked to viral infections, certain medications, or genetic factors.

- Hypertrophic cardiomyopathy: In this type, the heart muscle thickens abnormally, particularly in the septum (the wall separating the ventricles). This thickening can obstruct blood flow and make it harder for the heart to fill with blood. While often inherited, hypertrophic cardiomyopathy can also develop later in life.

- Restrictive cardiomyopathy: This type is characterized by stiffening of the heart muscle, making it difficult for the ventricles to relax and fill with blood. It can arise from various causes, including certain diseases that infiltrate the heart muscle, iron overload, or radiation therapy.

Symptoms of cardiomyopathy can vary depending on the type and severity, but may include fatigue, shortness of breath, chest pain, and swelling in the ankles and feet. Early diagnosis and treatment are crucial for managing cardiomyopathy and preventing complications like heart failure and arrhythmias.

Congenital Heart Defects: A Threat from the Start

Sometimes, the heart's structure may develop abnormally before birth. These congenital heart defects can range from mild to severe, affecting blood flow through the heart in various ways. Some common congenital heart defects include:

- Septal defects: These involve holes in the walls separating the heart chambers, allowing blood to flow abnormally between them.

- Valve defects: Babies can be born with heart valves that are malformed or narrowed, hindering proper blood flow.

- Heart malformations: These encompass various structural abnormalities, such as underdeveloped heart chambers or abnormal connections between blood vessels.

The symptoms of congenital heart defects also depend on the specific type and severity. In some cases, there might be no noticeable symptoms, while others may experience difficulty breathing, fatigue, or bluish discoloration of the skin (cyanosis).

Fortunately, significant advancements have been made in diagnosing and treating congenital heart defects. Many children born with heart defects can lead healthy lives with proper medical intervention, which may involve medications, catheter procedures, or open-heart surgery.

Unveiling the Untold Truths: A Call to Action

By exploring these "untold truths" about heart disease, we move beyond the singular image of blocked arteries. We recognize the multifaceted nature of this condition and the various ways it can threaten our well-being. This knowledge empowers us to take proactive steps towards prevention. Here are some key takeaways:

- Maintain a healthy lifestyle – a balanced diet, regular exercise, and managing weight are crucial for overall heart health.

- Control risk factors – address conditions like high blood pressure, high cholesterol, and diabetes, which can contribute to heart disease development.

- Know your family history – being aware of a family history of heart disease can help you identify your risk factors and take preventive measures.

- Schedule regular checkups – don't wait for symptoms to appear. Regular checkups and screenings can help detect heart disease early on, enabling timely intervention.

2.2 Beyond Blockages: Exploring Other Cardiovascular Conditions (e.g., Heart Failure, Arrhythmias)

Heart disease, the leading cause of death globally, often shrouds itself in a veil of misconceptions. When it comes to symptoms, the classic image of clutching your chest in pain dominates the narrative. But the reality is far more nuanced. Many heart conditions can progress silently, with subtle signs easily dismissed or attributed to other causes.

This lack of awareness can lead to delayed diagnosis and potentially life-threatening consequences.

Myth Busters: Dismantling Misconceptions about Heart Disease Symptoms

Let's debunk some common myths about heart disease symptoms, empowering you to recognize the silent threats lurking beneath the surface.

Myth #1: Only a crushing chest pain signifies a heart attack.

The Hollywood portrayal of a heart attack – a sudden, agonizing pain radiating down the left arm – is not always accurate. While chest pain is a common symptom, it can manifest in various ways:

* A squeezing, pressure, or tightness in the chest

* A burning or aching sensation in the chest

* Discomfort that travels to the arm, jaw, shoulder, or back

For some individuals, particularly women and diabetics, chest pain might be absent altogether. They might experience symptoms like:

* Shortness of breath, especially at rest or with exertion

* Fatigue and unusual tiredness

* Nausea, vomiting, or indigestion

* Lightheadedness, dizziness, or fainting

* Sweating

It's crucial to remember that these symptoms can also be caused by other conditions. However, if you experience any of them, particularly if they are persistent or worsening, don't hesitate to seek immediate medical attention. Early intervention can significantly improve outcomes in the event of a heart attack.

Myth #2: Heart disease only affects older adults.

While the risk of heart disease increases with age, it's a misconception that it's solely an oldie's concern. Younger adults can also be susceptible, especially if they have risk factors like high blood pressure, high cholesterol, diabetes, or a family history of heart disease. Additionally, certain lifestyle choices like smoking, unhealthy diet, and physical inactivity significantly contribute to the risk at any age.

Myth #3: If I feel fine, my heart must be healthy.

The silent nature of heart disease is its biggest threat. Many conditions, like coronary artery disease, can progress for years without any noticeable symptoms. This highlights the importance of preventive measures and regular checkups, even if you feel seemingly healthy. Early detection allows for timely intervention, potentially preventing complications and improving quality of life.

Beyond the Chest: Recognizing the Spectrum of Heart Disease Symptoms

As we saw earlier, heart disease encompasses a variety of conditions, each with its own set of potential symptoms. Here are some additional signs to be mindful of:

Heart failure: This can cause shortness of breath, particularly when lying down, fatigue, swelling in the ankles and feet, and rapid weight gain due to fluid buildup.

Arrhythmias: Depending on the type of arrhythmia, you might experience heart palpitations (feeling like your heart is racing or fluttering), chest pain, dizziness, or lightheadedness.

Heart valve disease: Symptoms can vary depending on the severity and type of valve dysfunction, but may include fatigue, shortness of breath, chest pain, or heart palpitations.

The Power of Early Detection: Why Every Beat Counts

Early detection is the cornerstone of successful heart disease management. By recognizing the subtle signs and seeking professional evaluation, you empower yourself to take charge of your heart health. Here's why early detection matters:

Improved treatment outcomes: Early intervention allows for treatments like medication, lifestyle modifications, or minimally invasive procedures to be more effective, potentially preventing complications and improving long-term prognosis.

Reduced risk of complications: Early diagnosis can help prevent heart failure, stroke, and other serious consequences associated with heart disease.

Enhanced quality of life: By managing heart disease effectively, you can maintain an active and fulfilling life for years to come.

Taking Action: Your Role in Early Detection

Here are some essential steps you can take to promote early detection of heart disease:

Know your family history: Understanding your risk factors based on your family lineage is crucial. Discuss any history of heart disease with your doctor.

Schedule regular checkups: Don't wait for symptoms to appear. Regular checkups allow your doctor to monitor your blood pressure, cholesterol levels, and overall heart health.

Maintain a healthy lifestyle: A balanced diet, regular exercise, and managing weight are essential for preventing heart disease.

Be mindful of your body: Pay attention to any changes in your health, even seemingly minor ones. If you experience any of the symptoms mentioned earlier, don't hesitate to consult your doctor.

CHAPTER THREE

THE UNTAPPED RISK FACTORS: BEYOND CHOLESTEROL

"Cholesterol – the silent villain!" This familiar refrain has dominated the heart health narrative for decades. While high cholesterol levels undoubtedly contribute to heart disease risk, the story is far more complex. Recent research has unveiled a spectrum of "untapped" risk factors lurking beneath the surface, influencing the health of your heart in surprising ways. By delving deeper into these often-overlooked factors, we can gain a more comprehensive understanding of heart health and take a holistic approach to prevention.

Beyond the Numbers Game: Unveiling the Nuances of Cholesterol

Let's begin by deconstructing the "cholesterol myth." Cholesterol itself isn't inherently bad. It's a waxy substance produced by the liver and found in certain foods.

It plays a vital role in various bodily functions, including cell membrane formation and hormone production. However, the problem arises when the balance between different types of cholesterol goes awry.

There are two main types of cholesterol to consider:

- LDL (low-density lipoprotein): Often referred to as "bad" cholesterol, LDL transports cholesterol particles throughout the bloodstream. When LDL levels are high, these particles can accumulate on the inner walls of arteries, forming plaque. Over time, this plaque buildup can narrow the arteries (atherosclerosis), restricting blood flow to the heart and increasing the risk of heart attack or stroke.

- HDL (high-density lipoprotein): This is the "good" cholesterol. HDL acts like a scavenger, picking up excess cholesterol particles from the bloodstream and transporting them back to the liver for disposal. Having healthy levels of HDL helps protect against plaque buildup.

The risk of heart disease isn't solely determined by total cholesterol levels. It's crucial to consider the ratio of LDL to HDL. A high LDL-to-HDL ratio indicates a greater risk of plaque buildup and heart disease. Additionally, a specific type of cholesterol called Lp(a) has recently emerged as a potential risk factor. Lp(a) is a more aggressive form of LDL and may contribute to plaque buildup even at "normal" LDL levels.

The Untapped Threats: A Wider Web of Risk Factors

While cholesterol remains a significant player, a multitude of other factors can influence heart health. Here are some often-underestimated culprits:

Chronic Inflammation: Inflammation, a natural immune response, can become chronic due to various factors like obesity, smoking, or a diet high in processed foods. Chronic inflammation can damage blood vessels and contribute to atheroma formation.

Sleep Apnea: This sleep disorder disrupts breathing patterns, leading to oxygen deprivation during sleep. This can damage the blood vessels and increase the risk of heart disease.

Stress: Chronic stress elevates stress hormones like cortisol, which can raise blood pressure and negatively impact heart health.

Environmental Toxins: Exposure to certain environmental toxins, like air pollution or heavy metals, can damage blood vessels and contribute to heart disease risk.

Gut Microbiome: Emerging research suggests the gut microbiome, the community of microorganisms living in our gut, may play a role in heart health. An imbalance in gut bacteria may contribute to inflammation and other processes linked to heart disease.

Social Determinants of Health: Social factors like poverty, lack of access to healthcare, and social isolation can significantly impact heart health. These factors can create chronic stress and limit access to health resources.

Untangling the Web: A Holistic Approach to Heart Health

Understanding these diverse risk factors empowers us to take a more comprehensive approach to safeguarding our hearts. Here's how you can weave a tapestry of heart-healthy habits:

Maintain a Balanced Diet: Focus on a diet rich in fruits, vegetables, whole grains, and lean protein. Limit saturated and trans fats, cholesterol, and added sodium. Consider incorporating foods rich in omega-3 fatty acids, found in fatty fish, which can help improve HDL levels.

Manage Weight: Excess weight puts additional strain on your heart. Aim for a healthy weight through a combination of a balanced diet and regular physical activity.

Prioritize Quality Sleep: Aim for 7-8 hours of quality sleep each night. If you suspect you might have sleep apnea, consult your doctor for diagnosis and treatment.

Manage Stress: Develop healthy coping mechanisms for stress, such as exercise, yoga, meditation, or spending time in nature.

Limit Alcohol Consumption: Excessive alcohol consumption can raise blood pressure and contribute to heart disease risk.

Don't Smoke: Smoking is one of the leading risk factors for heart disease. Quitting smoking is one of the most significant steps you can take for your heart health.

Regular Exercise: Engage in regular physical activity, aiming for at least 150 minutes of moderate-intensity exercise or 75 minutes of vigorous-intensity exercise per week.

Manage Existing Conditions: If you have conditions like high blood pressure, diabetes, or high cholesterol, work with your doctor to manage them effectively. This can significantly reduce your overall risk of heart disease.

Know Your Numbers: Regularly monitor your blood pressure, cholesterol levels, and blood sugar (if you have diabetes). This allows for early detection of any concerning changes and timely intervention.

Build a Strong Support System: Surround yourself with positive and supportive people who encourage healthy lifestyle choices.

Become an Advocate for Your Health: Be proactive in your healthcare. Ask questions, voice your concerns, and work collaboratively with your doctor to develop a personalized heart-healthy plan.

The Final Stitch: Weaving a Heart-Healthy Future

By acknowledging the "untapped" risk factors and adopting a holistic approach, we can empower ourselves to become active participants in safeguarding our hearts. Remember, heart disease isn't an inevitable fate. By taking charge of your lifestyle choices, managing existing conditions, and working with your doctor, you can significantly reduce your risk and weave a future rich with vibrant health.

3.1 The Inflammation Connection: How It Impacts Heart Health

Imagine a fire smoldering beneath the surface, silently wreaking havoc. This analogy aptly describes chronic inflammation, a hidden threat lurking within the body and playing a significant role in the development of heart disease. While inflammation is a natural, short-term response to injury or infection, when it becomes chronic and persists for extended periods, it can damage healthy tissues and contribute to various health problems, including heart disease.

The Fire Within: Unveiling the Link Between Inflammation and Heart Disease

The link between chronic inflammation and heart disease is a complex dance between the immune system, blood vessels, and the buildup of plaque in the arteries. Here's how it unfolds:

The Trigger: Chronic inflammation can arise from various factors like obesity, a diet high in processed foods and sugary drinks, smoking, and even certain gut bacteria imbalances. These triggers activate the immune system, leading to the release of inflammatory chemicals called cytokines.

A Battlefield Within: Cytokines, meant to fight infection or injury, can become problematic when chronically elevated. They can damage the inner lining of blood vessels, making them more susceptible to plaque buildup.

Fueling the Fire: Damaged blood vessels become sticky, attracting inflammatory cells and cholesterol particles. This accumulation gradually forms plaque, narrowing the arteries (atherosclerosis).

The Culmination: As plaque builds up, it can restrict blood flow to the heart, increasing the risk of angina (chest pain) and heart attack. In severe cases, a complete blockage can occur, triggering a heart attack and potentially leading to heart muscle death.

Beyond the Arteries: The Broader Impact of Inflammation

Chronic inflammation's impact extends beyond the arteries. It can also:

- Increase blood clotting risk: This can further elevate the risk of heart attack and stroke.

- Impair the function of the heart muscle: Chronic inflammation can weaken the heart muscle, hindering its ability to pump blood effectively and potentially contributing to heart failure.

- Disrupt blood sugar control: Chronic inflammation can impair the body's ability to regulate blood sugar levels, increasing the risk of type 2 diabetes, another significant risk factor for heart disease.

Extinguishing the Flames: Practical Tips to Reduce Inflammation

The good news is that chronic inflammation isn't an unyielding foe. By incorporating these evidence-based strategies, you can dampen the flames and promote a calmer, healthier internal environment:

Embrace an Anti-Inflammatory Diet: Focus on a diet rich in fruits, vegetables, whole grains, and lean protein. These foods are packed with antioxidants and other anti-inflammatory compounds. Conversely, limit processed foods, sugary drinks, refined carbohydrates, and unhealthy fats, as these can exacerbate inflammation.

Befriend Omega-3 Fatty Acids: Include omega-3 fatty acids, found in fatty fishlike salmon, tuna, and sardines, or flaxseeds and walnuts, in your diet. Omega-3s have potent anti-inflammatory properties.

Spice Up Your Life: Certain spices like turmeric, ginger, and garlic possess anti-inflammatory properties. Experiment with incorporating these into your meals for added flavor and health benefits.

Move Your Body Regularly: Exercise is a natural anti-inflammatory. Aim for at least 150 minutes of moderate-intensity exercise or 75 minutes of vigorous-intensity exercise per week. Even small bouts of daily activity can make a difference.

Manage Stress: Chronic stress can worsen inflammation. Find healthy ways to manage stress, such as yoga, meditation, deep breathing exercises, or spending time in nature.

Prioritize Sleep: Aim for 7-8 hours of quality sleep each night. Poor sleep can disrupt your body's natural anti-inflammatory mechanisms.

Consider Supplements: Consult your doctor about the potential benefits of anti-inflammatory supplements like fish oil or curcumin. However, remember that supplements shouldn't replace a healthy lifestyle.

Don't Smoke: Smoking is a major inflammatory trigger. Quitting smoking is one of the most significant steps you can take to reduce inflammation and improve your overall heart health.

Building a Fire Wall: Maintaining a Healthy Microbiome

Emerging research sheds light on the potential role of the gut microbiome, the trillions of microorganisms residing in our gut, in influencing inflammation and heart health. An imbalance in gut bacteria can contribute to chronic inflammation. Here's what you can do to nurture a healthy gut microbiome:

Eat a Fiber-Rich Diet: Fiber acts as a prebiotic, feeding the good bacteria in your gut.

Consider Probiotics: Probiotics are live bacteria found in fermented foods like yogurt and kimchi or in supplement form. They can help replenish your gut with beneficial bacteria.

Working with Your Doctor: A Collaborative Approach

While these strategies can significantly reduce inflammation, it's crucial to work collaboratively with your doctor. They can assess your individual risk factors and underlying health conditions. They can also:

- Monitor inflammatory markers: Blood tests can measure certain markers of inflammation, such as C-reactive protein (CRP) and interleukin-6 (IL-6). Monitoring these levels can help assess the effectiveness of your anti-inflammatory efforts.

- Address underlying conditions: If a specific condition, like obesity or an autoimmune disease, is contributing to chronic inflammation, treating the underlying issue can significantly reduce inflammation and improve your overall health.

- Develop a personalized plan: There's no "one-size-fits-all" approach to managing inflammation. Your doctor can work with you to create a personalized plan that incorporates dietary changes, exercise recommendations, stress management techniques, and, if necessary, medications to effectively manage chronic inflammation and protect your heart health.

The Power of Prevention: A Proactive Approach to Heart Health

By understanding the link between chronic inflammation and heart disease, you can take a proactive approach to safeguarding your heart. By incorporating anti-inflammatory strategies into your lifestyle and working collaboratively with your doctor, you can extinguish the flames of inflammation, reduce your risk of heart disease, and pave the way for a healthier, more vibrant future.

3.2 A Gut Feeling: The Microbiome and its Link to Cardiovascular Issues

For decades, the gut microbiome – the vast ecosystem of trillions of microorganisms residing within our intestines – has primarily been associated with digestion and nutrient absorption. However, recent scientific discoveries are unveiling a fascinating truth: the gut microbiome plays a surprisingly significant role in heart health. This emerging field of research holds immense promise for revolutionizing our understanding of heart disease prevention and treatment.

A Universe Within: Unveiling the Gut Microbiome

Imagine a bustling metropolis within your digestive system. This metropolis, teeming with trillions of bacterial citizens, is your gut microbiome. These microbial residents, encompassing a staggering variety of species, perform a multitude of tasks crucial for health. They break down complex carbohydrates, synthesize essential vitamins, and even help train our immune system.

The composition of this gut microbiome is unique to each individual and can be influenced by various factors, including diet, lifestyle choices, and even genetics. When the gut microbiome is balanced and diverse, with a healthy majority of beneficial bacteria, it thrives in a symbiotic relationship with its human host, promoting overall well-being. However, an imbalance in this ecosystem, with an overgrowth of harmful bacteria, can have detrimental consequences, including heightened susceptibility to various health problems, including heart disease.

The Gut-Heart Connection: A Two-Way Street

The gut and the heart, seemingly distant organs, are surprisingly interconnected. This communication highway is facilitated by the gut-brain axis, a complex network involving the nervous system, hormones, and the immune system. Here's a glimpse into how the gut microbiome can influence heart health:

Metabolite Production: Gut bacteria ferment dietary fibers and other undigested carbohydrates, producing metabolites like short-chain fatty acids (SCFAs). These SCFAs can influence blood pressure, cholesterol levels, and inflammation – all key players in heart disease development.

Immune System Modulation: The gut microbiome plays a crucial role in training and regulating the immune system. An imbalance in gut bacteria can lead to chronic, low-grade inflammation, which is a significant risk factor for heart disease.

Gut Permeability: A healthy gut lining acts as a barrier, preventing harmful substances and bacteria from leaking into the bloodstream. However, an unhealthy gut microbiome can contribute to increased gut permeability, allowing these elements to enter the bloodstream and potentially trigger inflammation throughout the body.

The Untold Story: How Gut Bacteria Can Impact Heart Disease Risk

Research suggests that an imbalance in gut bacteria may be associated with various heart disease risk factors:

Atherosclerosis: Certain gut bacteria may contribute to the formation of plaque in the arteries, a hallmark of atherosclerosis.

High Blood Pressure: An altered gut microbiome has been linked to elevated blood pressure, a major risk factor for heart disease.

High Cholesterol: Studies suggest the gut microbiome may influence cholesterol levels and metabolism, potentially impacting heart disease risk.

Cultivating a Heart-Healthy Gut: Dietary Strategies for a Balanced Microbiome

The good news is that you can nurture a healthy gut microbiome and potentially reduce your risk of heart disease through dietary modifications. Here are some key strategies:

Embrace Fiber-Rich Foods: Dietary fiber, found in fruits, vegetables, whole grains, and legumes, acts as a prebiotic, providing nourishment for the beneficial bacteria in your gut. By feeding these good bacteria, you help them thrive and maintain a balanced gut ecosystem.

Befriend Fermented Foods: Fermented foods like yogurt, kimchi, kefir, and kombucha are rich in probiotics – live bacteria with health benefits. Introducing these foods into your diet can help replenish your gut with beneficial bacterial strains.

Limit Processed Foods and Added Sugars: Processed foods and added sugars can disrupt the delicate balance of gut bacteria. Opt for whole, unprocessed foods whenever possible, and limit sugary drinks and snacks.

Consider Prebiotics: Prebiotics are non-digestible carbohydrates that selectively promote the growth and activity of beneficial bacteria. Foods like chicory root, Jerusalem artichokes, and garlic are good sources of prebiotics.

Building a Diverse Microbiome: Exploring Additional Strategies

Beyond dietary changes, other lifestyle practices can also promote a healthy gut microbiome:

- Manage Stress: Chronic stress can negatively impact gut health. Techniques like yoga, meditation, and deep breathing can help manage stress and promote a balanced gut environment.
- Prioritize Sleep: Aim for 7-8 hours of quality sleep each night. Sleep disturbances can disrupt gut bacteria composition.

- Exercise Regularly: Regular physical activity, even moderate-intensity exercise, can positively influence gut microbiome diversity.

Working with Your Doctor: A Collaborative Approach to Gut Health

While these strategies can significantly promote a healthy gut microbiome, it's crucial to collaborate with your doctor. They can:

Assess your individual needs: Based on your health history and risk factors, your doctor can guide you on the most appropriate dietary modifications and lifestyle changes to promote a gut microbiome beneficial for your heart health.

- Recommend prebiotic or probiotic supplements: In some cases, your doctor might recommend specific prebiotic or probiotic supplements to target imbalances in your gut bacteria. However, it's essential to remember that supplements should complement, not replace, a healthy diet and lifestyle.

- Address underlying conditions: If you have a digestive disorder like irritable bowel syndrome (IBS) or inflammatory bowel disease (IBD), managing these conditions can significantly improve your gut health and potentially reduce your risk of heart disease.

- Monitor progress: Through stool tests or other diagnostic tools, your doctor can monitor the composition of your gut microbiome over time, allowing them to adjust your personalized plan as needed.

The Future of Gut Health: Personalized Medicine and Beyond

The field of gut microbiome research is rapidly evolving. Scientists are exploring the potential of personalized medicine approaches tailored to an individual's unique gut bacterial makeup. This could involve targeted prebiotics, probiotics, or even fecal microbiota transplants (FMTs) to restore a healthy gut ecosystem and potentially prevent or manage various health conditions, including heart disease.

Empowering Your Heart Health: A Journey of Discovery

The link between the gut microbiome and heart health is a fascinating and complex story still being written. However, the current research offers a compelling message: by nurturing a diverse and healthy gut microbiome, you can take a proactive step towards safeguarding your heart. Embrace a diet rich in fiber and fermented foods, minimize processed foods and added sugars, prioritize stress management and sleep, and engage in regular physical activity. By working collaboratively with your doctor, you can unlock the potential of your gut microbiome and empower yourself on a journey towards a healthier, heart-stronger you.

CHAPTER FOUR

THE STRESS PARADOX: HOW EMOTIONAL WELLBEING IMPACTS YOUR HEART

"A merry heart doeth good like a medicine, but a broken spirit drieth the bones," proclaims Proverbs 17:22.

This ancient wisdom resonates deeply with a truth increasingly recognized by modern medicine: emotional well-being has a profound impact on heart health. The stress paradox, however, unveils a complex dance between our emotions and the well-being of our hearts. While stress is often villainized as a heart health culprit, the reality is more nuanced. Understanding this paradox empowers us to harness the positive aspects of emotional well-being and mitigate the detrimental effects of chronic stress.

The Dark Side of Stress: How It Can Threaten Your Heart

Stress, a natural response to perceived threats or challenges, is a double-edged sword. In the short term, it can be beneficial, triggering the "fight-or-flight" response, which prepares the body for action. This surge of hormones, like adrenaline and cortisol, temporarily increases heart rate, blood pressure, and blood sugar to meet the perceived threat. However, when stress becomes chronic and unrelenting, it can wreak havoc on your heart in several ways:

Elevated Blood Pressure: Chronic stress can lead to sustained high blood pressure, a major risk factor for heart disease. The constant activation of the fight-or-flight response keeps blood pressure elevated, putting a strain on the heart and increasing the risk of heart attack or stroke.

Increased Inflammation: Stress can trigger the release of inflammatory chemicals in the body. Chronic inflammation damages blood vessels and contributes to the buildup of plaque in the arteries (atherosclerosis), which narrows the arteries and further increases the risk of heart attack and stroke.

Unhealthy Lifestyle Choices: When stressed, you might be more likely to engage in unhealthy behaviors like smoking, overeating, or physical inactivity, all of which contribute to heart disease risk.

Disrupted Sleep: Stress can significantly disrupt sleep patterns, leading to sleep deprivation. This can further elevate blood pressure, impair heart function, and increase the risk of heart disease.

The Sunny Side Up: The Positive Power of Emotions

The stress paradox reveals a surprising truth: not all stress is detrimental to heart health. Positive emotions like happiness, hope, and gratitude can have a surprisingly protective effect on the heart. Here's how:

Improved Blood Pressure: Studies suggest that positive emotions can lead to lower blood pressure, reducing the strain on the heart. Laughter, for example, can have a temporary vasodilatory effect, relaxing blood vessels and lowering blood pressure.

Enhanced Social Connections: Strong social connections and feelings of belonging can contribute to a sense of well-being, reducing stress and potentially lowering the risk of heart disease.

Healthier Lifestyle Choices: When you feel happy and optimistic, you're more likely to engage in healthy behaviors like regular exercise and a balanced diet, both of which benefit heart health.

Stress Resilience: Positive emotions can enhance your ability to cope with stress in a healthy way, making you more resilient in the face of challenges and reducing the negative impact of chronic stress on your heart.

Beyond Black and White: The Spectrum of Emotional Well-being

The relationship between stress and heart health isn't a simple binary. Individual differences play a significant role. Some people are naturally more susceptible to the negative effects of stress, while others seem to have a higher tolerance. Additionally, the type of stressor matters. Chronic work-related stress can have a greater detrimental impact than the temporary stress of public speaking.

Unmasking the Hidden Culprit: When "Good" Stress Turns Bad

The stress paradox also highlights the distinction between acute stress and chronic stress. Acute stress, as experienced during a challenging presentation or a competitive game, can be motivating and energizing. However, when this acute stress becomes chronic and unrelenting, it can turn detrimental. Recognizing the warning signs of chronic stress, such as persistent anxiety, fatigue, irritability, or difficulty sleeping, is crucial.

Embracing Emotional Intelligence: Cultivating a Heart-Healthy Mindset

By understanding the stress paradox, we can empower ourselves to cultivate a heart-healthy emotional well-being. Here are some strategies to embrace emotional intelligence and manage stress effectively:

Identify Your Stress Triggers: Recognizing the situations or events that trigger stress in you is the first step towards managing it.

Develop Coping Mechanisms: Develop healthy coping mechanisms to deal with stress, such as relaxation techniques like deep breathing or meditation, regular exercise, spending time in nature, or engaging in hobbies you enjoy.

Build Strong Social Connections: Foster strong social connections with friends and family. Strong social support can be a powerful buffer against stress and contribute to overall well-being.

Practice Gratitude: Cultivate an attitude of gratitude. Focusing on the positive aspects of your life can enhance happiness and reduce stress.

4.1 The Biological Link: From Stress Hormones to Physical Changes

Imagine a well-rehearsed orchestra, each section playing in harmony. This is how the body functions under normal circumstances. However, introduce a chronic, nagging stressor, and the music turns discordant, potentially leading to a symphony of health problems, including heart disease. This subchapter dig into the biological link between chronic stress, stress hormones, and the physical changes that elevate your risk of heart disease.

The Fight-or-Flight Response: A Necessary Adaptation

Stress, a natural response to perceived threats or challenges, is a survival mechanism inherited from our ancestors. When faced with danger, the body initiates the "fight-or-flight" response, a cascade of events designed to prepare for immediate action. This response is orchestrated by the hypothalamus, a tiny control center in the brain, which triggers the release of hormones like adrenaline and cortisol from the adrenal glands.

The Hormonal Symphony: Adrenaline and Cortisol Take Center Stage

Adrenaline: This hormone acts like a conductor, rapidly increasing heart rate, blood pressure, and blood sugar levels. This surge of energy prepares the body for immediate action, be it fight or flight. In the short term, this response is beneficial, allowing us to escape danger.

Cortisol: Often referred to as the "stress hormone," cortisol plays a vital role in managing stress. It increases blood sugar levels to provide readily available energy, suppresses non-essential functions like digestion, and enhances alertness. However, these effects are meant to be temporary.

When the Music Gets Stuck: Chronic Stress and the Hormonal Imbalance

In today's world, stressors are often chronic and unrelenting – deadlines, financial pressures, relationship difficulties. This constant activation of the fight-or-flight response keeps the hormonal orchestra playing a stressful tune, leading to several detrimental effects on your heart health:

Elevated Blood Pressure: Chronic stress keeps adrenaline and cortisol levels elevated. These hormones constrict blood vessels and increase heart rate, leading to sustained high blood pressure. This persistent strain on the heart weakens it over time and increases the risk of heart attack and stroke.

Endothelial Dysfunction: The endothelium, the inner lining of your blood vessels, plays a crucial role in regulating blood pressure and preventing blood clots. Chronic stress can damage the endothelium, making it less elastic and more prone to inflammation. This dysfunction further contributes to high blood pressure and increases the risk of atherosclerosis, the buildup of plaque in the arteries.

Metabolic Disruption: Chronically elevated cortisol levels can disrupt your body's ability to regulate blood sugar levels, potentially leading to insulin resistance and type 2 diabetes, another significant risk factor for heart disease.

Inflammation on High: Chronic stress triggers the release of inflammatory chemicals in the body. This persistent inflammation damages blood vessels, contributes to plaque buildup, and increases the overall risk of heart disease.

The Vicious Cycle: How Stress Begets More Stress

Unfortunately, the impact of chronic stress on heart health becomes a vicious cycle. The physical changes it induces – high blood pressure, impaired blood flow, and potential heart damage – can further heighten anxiety and stress, perpetuating the hormonal imbalance and increasing the risk of heart problems.

Beyond the Symphony: Additional Consequences of Chronic Stress

Chronic stress can wreak havoc on your overall health beyond its impact on the heart. It can weaken your immune system, making you more susceptible to infections; disrupt sleep patterns, leading to fatigue and decreased energy levels; and even contribute to mood disorders like anxiety and depression.

Breaking the Cycle: Strategies for Managing Chronic Stress

The good news is that you're not powerless against chronic stress. By incorporating these strategies, you can become the conductor of your own well-being and rewrite the stressful symphony into a heart-healthy masterpiece:

Identify Your Stress Triggers: Recognizing the situations or events that trigger stress in you is the first step towards managing it.

Develop Healthy Coping Mechanisms: Develop healthy ways to cope with stress. Techniques like relaxation techniques (deep breathing, meditation), regular exercise, spending time in nature, or engaging in hobbies you enjoy can all help alleviate stress.

Prioritize Sleep: Aim for 7-8 hours of quality sleep each night. Chronic sleep deprivation can worsen stress and exacerbate its negative effects on your heart.

Build Strong Social Connections: Social support is a powerful buffer against stress. Foster strong relationships with friends and family, and don't hesitate to seek professional help from a therapist or counselor if needed.

Working with Your Doctor: A Collaborative Approach

While these strategies empower you to manage stress, it's crucial to work collaboratively with your doctor. They can:

- Assess your individual risk factors: Based on your health history and risk factors, your doctor can tailor a stress management plan that works best for you.

- Recommend additional support: If necessary, your doctor might recommend additional support, such as:

- Cognitive-behavioral therapy (CBT): This form of therapy can help you identify and change negative thought patterns that contribute to stress.

- Medication: In some cases, your doctor might prescribe medication to manage anxiety or depression, which can often co-occur with chronic stress.

The Power of Mindfulness: Cultivating Inner Peace

Mindfulness practices, which involve focusing your attention on the present moment without judgment, can be remarkably effective in managing stress and promoting relaxation. Techniques like meditation, yoga, and mindful breathing can help you become more aware of your stress triggers and responses, allowing you to develop healthier coping mechanisms.

The Final Note: A Heart-Healthy Harmony

By understanding the biological link between chronic stress, stress hormones, and their impact on heart health, you can take proactive steps to break the cycle of stress and cultivate a symphony of well-being. Remember, managing stress isn't about eliminating all challenges from your life. It's about learning to navigate them in a way that safeguards your heart and promotes overall health. Embrace healthy coping mechanisms, prioritize relaxation techniques, and work collaboratively with your doctor. By taking charge of your emotional well-being, you can rewrite the stressful symphony into a heart-healthy masterpiece, ensuring your heart continues to beat strong for years to come.

4.2 The Vicious Cycle: How Heart Disease Worsens Mental Health

Chronic stress, often dismissed as an inevitable part of modern life, casts a long shadow on our health, particularly heart health. Its impact isn't always immediate or dramatic, but the silent erosion it inflicts can have devastating consequences. This subchapter sifts into the real-life stories of individuals, showcasing how chronic stress manifests differently in their lives, ultimately affecting their heart health.

Tasha: The Workaholic Warrior

Tasha, a driven investment banker, thrives on the adrenaline rush of deadlines and high-pressure deals. Sleep is a luxury she rarely affords, replaced by late nights poring over spreadsheets and endless conference calls. While Tasha appears invincible on the surface, the constant pressure takes a toll. Her blood pressure remains stubbornly elevated, a warning sign ignored in the pursuit of professional success. The chronic stress also disrupts her sleep, leading to fatigue and difficulty concentrating. One morning, a crushing tightness in her chest sends her to the emergency room, where she receives a life-altering diagnosis: angina, a symptom of coronary heart disease. Tasha's relentless work ethic, fueled by chronic stress, had silently compromised her heart health.

Michael: The Bottled-Up Burden

Michael, a reserved accountant, internalizes his stress. He rarely expresses his anxieties, bottling them up inside. He finds solace in unhealthy habits - excessive sugar intake and a sedentary lifestyle. The chronic stress triggers low-grade inflammation in his body, further damaging his blood vessels. Over time, Michael develops prediabetes, a condition that raises his risk of heart disease. He experiences occasional chest pain, which he dismisses as indigestion, further delaying seeking medical attention. When a routine blood test reveals high cholesterol levels,

Michael is forced to confront the consequences of his unaddressed stress.

Emily: The Juggling Act

Emily, a single mother of two young children, juggles a demanding job with the relentless responsibilities of parenthood. Sleep deprivation becomes her norm, replaced by late-night diaper changes and early morning wake-up calls. The constant pressure and exhaustion leave her feeling overwhelmed and on edge. The chronic stress disrupts her eating habits, leading to a reliance on fast food for convenience. This unhealthy diet, coupled with minimal physical activity due to time constraints, puts a strain on her heart. During a routine check-up, Emily discovers she has borderline high blood pressure. Recognizing the need for change, she starts prioritizing self-care, incorporating stress management techniques and healthier meal choices into her hectic schedule.

The Common Thread: Stress and Heart Health

While Sarah, Michael, and Emily faced different stressors and exhibited various coping mechanisms, the underlying theme remains the same: chronic stress significantly impacted their heart health. Sarah's workaholism led to high blood pressure and coronary heart disease. Michael's internalized stress contributed to inflammation, prediabetes, and high cholesterol. Emily's juggling act resulted in poor dietary choices, lack of exercise, and borderline high blood pressure.

Beyond the Case Studies: Recognizing the Varied Faces of Stress

These case studies illustrate the diverse ways chronic stress can manifest and its detrimental impact on heart health. However, the impact of stress isn't universal. Here are some additional factors that influence how stress affects individuals:

- Personality: People with Type A personalities — characterized by competitiveness, impatience, and hostility – are more susceptible to the damaging effects of chronic stress.

- Social Support: Strong social connections can act as a buffer against stress. Conversely, social isolation can exacerbate its negative effects.

- Genetic Predisposition: Some individuals have a genetic predisposition to be more susceptible to the physical consequences of stress.

Unmasking the Hidden Culprit: When Physical Symptoms Point to Stress

Chronic stress doesn't always manifest as anxiety or emotional distress. In some cases, it can masquerade as physical symptoms, often leading to confusion and misdiagnosis. Here are some signs that chronic stress might be affecting your heart health:

- Unexplained fatigue: Persistent tiredness that doesn't improve with adequate sleep can be a sign of chronic stress and its impact on heart health.

- Headaches and muscle tension: Chronic stress can manifest as frequent headaches and muscle tension throughout the body.

- Sleep disturbances: Difficulty falling asleep, staying asleep, or experiencing restless sleep are common symptoms of chronic stress that can further worsen heart health.

- Changes in appetite: Stress can lead to either overeating or loss of appetite, contributing to unhealthy dietary choices and potentially increasing heart disease risk.

- Digestive issues: Chronic stress can disrupt the digestive system, leading to problems like constipation, diarrhea, and heartburn.

Breaking Free from the Grip of Stress: Strategies for a Heart-Healthy Lifestyle

The good news is that chronic stress isn't an inevitable sentence. By incorporating simple strategies into your daily life, you can effectively manage stress and protect your heart:

Identify Your Stress Triggers: The first step towards managing stress is recognizing the situations, events, or people that trigger your stress response. Are you a workaholic like Tasha, prone to neglecting sleep and self-care? Do you, like Michael, internalize stress and avoid expressing your anxieties? Perhaps you juggle multiple responsibilities like Emily, leading to a chaotic and high-pressure lifestyle. Once you pinpoint your specific stress triggers, you can begin to develop coping mechanisms to address them effectively.

Develop Healthy Coping Mechanisms: Instead of resorting to unhealthy habits like overeating or social isolation, cultivate healthy coping mechanisms to manage stress. Techniques like relaxation exercises (deep breathing, meditation, progressive muscle relaxation) can help calm your nervous system and promote feelings of well-being. Regular physical activity, even moderate exercise like brisk walking, can be a powerful stress reliever and benefit your heart health directly.

Prioritize Sleep: Chronic sleep deprivation exacerbates stress and weakens your heart. Aim for 7-8 hours of quality sleep each night. Develop a relaxing bedtime routine and create a sleep-conducive environment to ensure restful sleep.

Build Strong Social Connections: Social support is a powerful buffer against stress. Nurture relationships with friends and family who offer emotional support and a sense of belonging. Don't hesitate to seek professional help from a therapist or counselor if you need additional support in managing stress.

Practice Mindfulness: Mindfulness practices, which involve focusing your attention on the present moment without judgment, can be remarkably effective in managing stress and promoting relaxation. Whether it's meditation, yoga, or simply spending time in nature, incorporating mindfulness into your daily routine can help you become more aware of your stress triggers and responses, allowing you to develop healthier coping mechanisms.

Learn to Say No: Don't overload your schedule with unrealistic commitments. Saying no to additional responsibilities when you're already stretched thin is a crucial skill for managing stress and protecting your well-being. Prioritize self-care and ensure you have enough time to relax and recharge.

Working with Your Doctor: A Collaborative Approach

While these strategies empower you to manage stress, it's crucial to collaborate with your doctor. They can:

Assess your individual risk factors: Based on your health history, family history, and lifestyle habits, your doctor can assess your individual risk factors for heart disease. This allows them to tailor a stress management plan that works best for you.

Recommend additional support: If your stress levels are significantly impacting your well-being, your doctor might recommend additional support, such as cognitive-behavioral therapy (CBT). This form of therapy can help you identify and change negative thought patterns that contribute to stress and anxiety. In some cases, medication might be necessary to manage co-occurring conditions like depression that can worsen the impact of stress on your heart health.

The Untold Truth: It's All Connected

Chronic stress is more than just a feeling of being overwhelmed. It's a biological cascade with significant consequences for your heart health. The case studies presented here offer a glimpse into the diverse ways stress can manifest and its detrimental impact on the heart. By recognizing your stress triggers, developing healthy coping mechanisms, and working collaboratively with your doctor, you can break free from the grip of stress and cultivate a heart-healthy lifestyle. Remember, prioritizing your mental and emotional well-being is an essential part of safeguarding your physical health, especially your heart. Start incorporating these strategies into your daily life today and rewrite the story of stress, ensuring your heart continues to beat strong for years to come.

CHAPTER FIVE

BREAKING FREE: STRATEGIES FOR MANAGING STRESS AND ANXIETY

"The greatest weapon against stress is our ability to choose one thought over another," declares W. Clement Stone, a renowned motivational speaker.

This powerful statement underscores a fundamental truth: stress, while often perceived as an external force, can be significantly influenced by our internal choices and strategies. In the quest for a heart-healthy life, effectively managing stress and anxiety becomes an essential weapon in your arsenal. This chapter dig into practical strategies that empower you to break free from the grip of stress and cultivate a sense of calm and well-being.

The Duality of Stress and Anxiety: Understanding the Nuances

Stress and anxiety are often used interchangeably, but there are subtle distinctions. Stress is a natural response to perceived threats or challenges. It can be short-term, motivating us to take action and prepare for a presentation or exam. However, chronic stress, when left unmanaged, can morph into anxiety – a persistent feeling of worry or unease that disrupts daily life and negatively impacts both mental and physical health.

The Unseen Threat: How Stress and Anxiety Endanger Your Heart

Chronic stress and anxiety are more than just unpleasant feelings; they pose a significant threat to your heart health. Here's how:

Elevated Blood Pressure: Stress hormones like adrenaline and cortisol constrict blood vessels and increase heart rate, leading to sustained high blood pressure – a major risk factor for heart attack and stroke.

Endothelial Dysfunction: The endothelium, the inner lining of your blood vessels, plays a crucial role in regulating blood pressure and preventing blood clots. Chronic stress can damage the endothelium, making it less elastic and more prone to inflammation, further contributing to heart disease risk.

Metabolic Disruption: Chronically elevated cortisol levels can disrupt your body's ability to regulate blood sugar levels, potentially leading to insulin resistance and type 2 diabetes, another significant risk factor for heart disease.

Inflammation on High: Chronic stress triggers the release of inflammatory chemicals in the body. This persistent inflammation damages blood vessels, contributes to plaque buildup, and increases the overall risk of heart disease.

The Vicious Cycle: How Stress Begets More Stress

Unfortunately, the impact of chronic stress on heart health becomes a vicious cycle. The physical changes it induces – high blood pressure, impaired blood flow, and potential heart damage – can further heighten anxiety and stress, perpetuating the hormonal imbalance and increasing the risk of heart problems.

The Power of Choice: Embracing Strategies for Stress Management

The good news is that you're not powerless against stress and anxiety. By incorporating these strategies, you can become an active participant in your well-being and build resilience against chronic stress:

Identify Your Stress Triggers: The first step towards managing stress is recognizing the situations, events, or people that trigger your stress response. Are you prone to work overload, similar to Sarah from Chapter 4? Do you struggle with social anxieties, or do financial pressures keep you up at night? Once you pinpoint your specific stress triggers, you can begin to develop coping mechanisms to address them effectively.

Develop Healthy Coping Mechanisms: Instead of resorting to unhealthy habits like overeating or social isolation, cultivate healthy coping mechanisms to manage stress. Here are some powerful techniques to explore:

Relaxation Techniques: Practices like deep breathing, progressive muscle relaxation, and meditation can activate the body's relaxation response, counteracting the fight-or-flight response triggered by stress.

Regular Exercise: Physical activity is a potent stress reliever. Aim for at least 30 minutes of moderate-intensity exercise most days of the week. Brisk walking, swimming, cycling, or dancing are all excellent options.

Mindfulness Practices: Mindfulness techniques like meditation or yoga can help you become more aware of your thoughts and feelings without judgment. This increased self-awareness empowers you to respond to stress in a more mindful and constructive way.

Prioritize Sleep: Chronic sleep deprivation exacerbates stress and weakens your heart. Aim for 7-8 hours of quality sleep each night. Develop a relaxing bedtime routine and create a sleep-conducive environment to ensure restful sleep.

Build Strong Social Connections: Social support is a powerful buffer against stress. Nurture relationships with friends and family who offer emotional support and a sense of belonging. Don't hesitate to seek professional help from a therapist or counselor if you need additional support in managing stress.

Practice Gratitude: Cultivating an attitude of gratitude can significantly reduce stress and enhance well-being. Take time each day to reflect on the positive aspects of your life, big or small. Expressing gratitude can shift your focus away from stressors and promote a sense of calmness.

Learn to Say No: Don't overload your schedule with unrealistic commitments. Saying no to additional responsibilities when you're already stretched thin is a crucial skill for managing stress and protecting your well-being. Prioritize self-care and ensure you have enough time to relax and recharge. Saying no might feel uncomfortable initially, but it empowers you to set healthy boundaries and avoid the detrimental effects of chronic stress on your heart health.

Challenge Negative Thoughts: Stress and anxiety often fuel negative thought patterns. Challenge these self-defeating beliefs and replace them with more positive and realistic affirmations. Cognitive-behavioral therapy (CBT) can be a valuable tool in identifying and reframing negative thought patterns that contribute to stress and anxiety.

Practice Time Management: Feeling overwhelmed and behind schedule can be a significant stressor. Develop effective time management skills. Learn to prioritize tasks, delegate when possible, and create realistic to-do lists to avoid feeling constantly overloaded.

Engage in Activities You Enjoy: Make time for activities that bring you joy and relaxation. Whether it's reading, spending time in nature, listening to music, or pursuing hobbies, prioritize activities that help you de-stress and recharge.

Laughter is the Best Medicine: Laughter is a powerful antidote to stress. Watch a funny movie, spend time with people who make you laugh, or read humorous stories.

Laughter has been shown to lower stress hormones, elevate mood, and boost the immune system, all of which benefit your heart health.

Working with Your Doctor: A Collaborative Approach

While these strategies empower you to manage stress and anxiety, it's crucial to collaborate with your doctor. They can:

Assess your individual risk factors: Based on your health history, family history, and lifestyle habits, your doctor can assess your individual risk factors for heart disease. This allows them to tailor a stress management plan that works best for you.

Recommend additional support: If your stress levels are significantly impacting your well-being, your doctor might recommend additional support, such as cognitive-behavioral therapy (CBT) or medication. CBT can help you identify and change negative thought patterns that contribute to stress and anxiety. In some cases, medication might be necessary to manage co-occurring conditions like depression that can worsen the impact of stress on your heart health.

Building Resilience: Cultivating a Stress-Resistant Lifestyle

By incorporating these strategies into your daily life, you can build resilience against chronic stress and anxiety. Remember, stress management is an ongoing process. There will be times when stress levels rise, but by equipping yourself with a toolbox of healthy coping mechanisms, you can effectively navigate these challenges and safeguard your heart health. The more you prioritize stress management, the more empowered you become to cultivate a sense of calm and well-being, fostering a heart-healthy and fulfilling life.

5.1 Mind-Body Techniques for Relaxation: Meditation, Yoga, and Deep Breathing

Chronic stress and anxiety cast a long shadow on our heart health. However, nestled within us lies a wellspring of resilience: the mind-body connection. This subchapter jumps into powerful mind-body techniques like meditation, yoga, and deep breathing, equipping you with practical tools to manage stress, cultivate inner peace, and ultimately safeguard your heart.

Meditation: A Journey Within

Meditation, often shrouded in mystery, is a simple yet profound practice that cultivates mindfulness – the ability to focus your attention on the present moment without judgment. Here's a step-by-step guide for beginners to embark on their meditation journey:

Finding Your Sanctuary: Choose a quiet, comfortable space free from distractions. Dim the lights if desired, and ensure a comfortable temperature.

Assuming a Comfortable Posture: Sit upright in a chair with your feet flat on the floor or kneel on a cushion. Maintain a tall spine without feeling rigid, allowing for natural curves.

Closing Your Eyes (Optional): Gently close your eyes if you feel comfortable doing so. Alternatively, you can soften your gaze by focusing on a point on the floor a few feet in front of you.

Anchoring Your Breath: Begin by bringing your attention to your breath. Feel the natural rise and fall of your chest and abdomen with each inhale and exhale. Don't try to control your breath; simply observe it.

Wandering Thoughts: It's Okay: Inevitably, your mind will wander. This is normal. Acknowledge the thought without judgment and gently guide your attention back to your breath. Think of your mind like a curious puppy – it might stray, but you can always gently bring it back.

The Art of Non-Judgment: As thoughts, emotions, or bodily sensations arise, observe them with a sense of curiosity and acceptance. Don't judge yourself for having these experiences.

Be Kind to Yourself: Start with short meditation sessions, even just 5 minutes. Gradually increase the duration as you become more comfortable. Remember, consistency is key. The goal isn't to achieve a state of perfect emptiness; it's about cultivating awareness and calmness.

Yoga: The Harmony of Body and Mind

Yoga offers a holistic approach to well-being, combining physical postures (asanas), breathing exercises (pranayama), and meditation. Here's a basic introduction to some beginner-friendly yoga poses that promote relaxation and stress reduction:

Child's Pose (Balasana): Kneel on the floor with your toes together and knees hip-width apart. Sit back on your heels and rest your forehead on the mat, extending your arms out in front of you or alongside your body. Close your eyes and take slow, deep breaths.

Downward-Facing Dog (Adho Mukha Svanasana): Start on your hands and knees with your knees hip-width apart and hands shoulder-width apart. Push your hips back and up, straightening your legs as much as comfortably possible. Create a long line from your heels to your fingertips. Keep your head in line with your spine, gazing slightly back between your legs. Hold for a few breaths.

Cat-Cow Pose (Marjaryasana and Bitilasana): Begin on your hands and knees with your hands shoulder-width apart and knees hip-width apart. As you inhale, arch your back, dropping your belly towards the floor and looking up. As you exhale, round your back, tucking your chin to your chest and engaging your abdominal muscles. Flow between these movements in a synchronized breath.

Corpse Pose (Savasana): Lie flat on your back with your arms at your sides and palms facing up. Close your eyes and allow your entire body to relax. Focus on your breath and allow any tension to melt away. Hold for several minutes.

Deep Breathing: The Power of Simplicity

Deep breathing, a fundamental aspect of meditation and yoga, is a powerful tool for managing stress and anxiety in its own right. Here's how to practice deep breathing:

Find a Comfortable Position: Sit or lie down in a comfortable position with your back straight.

Engaging Your Diaphragm: Place one hand on your chest and the other on your abdomen. As you inhale slowly through your nose, feel your abdomen expand (not your chest) as your diaphragm contracts.

The Pause at the Top: Hold your breath briefly at the top of your inhale for a count of one.

Exhale Slowly: Exhale slowly and completely through your pursed lips, feeling your abdomen gently contract as your diaphragm relaxes.

Repeat and Relax: Aim for 5-10 repetitions of this complete breathing cycle. Focus on your breath and the sensations in your body. With each exhale, imagine releasing tension and stress.

Beyond the Basics: Exploring Additional Techniques

Meditation, yoga, and deep breathing are just the tip of the iceberg when it comes to mind-body techniques for stress management. Here are some additional options to explore:

Progressive Muscle Relaxation: This technique involves tensing and relaxing different muscle groups throughout your body, promoting a deep sense of relaxation.

Guided Imagery: Close your eyes and visualize a peaceful scene or experience, allowing it to evoke feelings of calm and serenity.

Mindfulness in Everyday Activities: Incorporate mindfulness into your daily routine. Focus on the present moment as you brush your teeth, wash the dishes, or take a walk. Pay attention to the sensations in your body and the details of your surroundings.

The Science Behind the Practice: How Mind-Body Techniques Benefit Your Heart

Mind-body techniques aren't just about feeling good in the moment. Research suggests they offer a range of benefits for your heart health:

Lowering Blood Pressure: Studies have shown that regular meditation practice can lead to a reduction in blood pressure, a significant risk factor for heart disease.

Reducing Inflammation: Mind-body techniques can help modulate the body's inflammatory response, which plays a role in the development of heart disease.

Improving Sleep Quality: Chronic stress often disrupts sleep patterns. Mind-body practices like meditation and yoga can promote better sleep, which is crucial for heart health.

Enhancing Emotional Regulation: These techniques can equip you with tools to manage stress and anxiety more effectively, leading to a calmer emotional state and reduced strain on your heart.

Cultivating a Sustainable Practice: Making Mind-Body Techniques a Habit

Integrating mind-body practices into your daily life requires commitment. Here are some tips for building a sustainable practice:

Start Small: Don't overwhelm yourself. Begin with short meditation sessions (5 minutes) or a few simple yoga poses. Gradually increase the duration and complexity as you become more comfortable.

Find a Routine: Schedule your practice into your daily routine, just like brushing your teeth or taking a shower. Consistency is key to reaping the long-term benefits.

Explore Different Techniques: Experiment with different mind-body practices to find what resonates most with you. There's no one-size-fits-all approach.

Be Patient: It takes time and practice to cultivate the mind-body connection. Don't get discouraged if you don't experience immediate results. The journey itself is valuable.

Seek Support: Join a meditation or yoga class for added motivation and guidance. There are also numerous online resources and apps available to help you on your journey.

The Untold Truth: The Power Lies Within

By harnessing the mind-body connection through techniques like meditation, yoga, and deep breathing, you become an active participant in your well-being. These practices are powerful tools for managing stress and anxiety, ultimately safeguarding your heart health. Remember, fostering inner peace and resilience is an ongoing process. Embrace the journey, and empower yourself to cultivate a heart-healthy and fulfilling life.

5.2 Cognitive Behavioral Therapy (CBT): Reshaping Thoughts for a Healthier Heart

Chronic stress and anxiety often stem from distorted thinking patterns. We magnify threats, minimize our coping abilities, and get caught in negative thought spirals. This subchapter sifts into Cognitive Behavioral Therapy (CBT), a powerful tool that empowers you to challenge these unhelpful thought patterns and cultivate a more balanced perspective, ultimately safeguarding your heart health.

Understanding CBT: Reshaping Your Thinking for a Calmer You

Developed by psychiatrist Aaron T. Beck, CBT is a form of psychotherapy that focuses on the connection between your thoughts, feelings, and behaviors. It operates on the principle that our thoughts and interpretations of situations significantly influence our emotional and physical responses. By modifying these thought patterns, we can effectively manage stress and anxiety.

How CBT Benefits Your Heart Health:

Chronic stress and anxiety, fueled by negative thought patterns, wreak havoc on your heart health. Here's how CBT can help:

Reduced Stress Hormones: CBT helps you identify and challenge negative thoughts that trigger the release of stress hormones like cortisol and adrenaline. By reframing these thoughts, you can lower stress hormone levels, easing the strain on your heart.

Improved Emotional Regulation: CBT equips you with tools to manage difficult emotions more effectively. This emotional regulation reduces the stress response and its negative impact on your cardiovascular system.

Enhanced Coping Mechanisms: CBT helps you develop healthy coping skills to navigate stressful situations. This reduces the anxiety response and promotes a calmer emotional state, benefiting your heart health.

Practical Exercises for Taming the Thought Monster:

CBT isn't just a passive therapy; it's an active process of self-discovery and thought modification. Here are some practical exercises you can incorporate into your daily life:

- The ABCs of CBT: This simple framework helps you identify the relationship between activating events, beliefs, consequences, and emotional and behavioral responses. Here's how it works:
- Activating Event: Identify the situation or trigger that evokes stress or anxiety.

- Beliefs: Pinpoint the thoughts and beliefs you have about the situation. Are they realistic or distorted?

- Consequences: Consider the emotional and physical consequences of your beliefs.

- Challenge & Reframe: Challenge the negative or unhelpful beliefs you identified. Can you reframe them into more realistic and empowering thoughts?

- The Thought Log: Maintain a thought log to track your negative thought patterns. Record the situation, your automatic thoughts, the emotions they trigger, and the evidence for and against those thoughts. This process helps you identify cognitive distortions and develop more balanced perspectives.

- Cognitive Restructuring Techniques: CBT employs various techniques to challenge and reframe negative thoughts. Here are a few examples:

- Dec catastrophizing: Don't jump to worst-case scenarios. Consider more realistic and positive outcomes.

- Identifying All-or-Nothing Thinking: Life isn't black and white. Challenge thoughts like "I have to be perfect" or "If I fail, it's all over."
- Spotlighting Labeling and Overgeneralization: Don't label yourself or situations based on a single event. Avoid overgeneralizations like "I always mess up."

Beyond the Exercises: Building a Sustainable CBT Practice

CBT is a valuable tool, but it requires consistent effort to see lasting results. Here are some tips for building a sustainable CBT practice:

Seek Professional Guidance: While these exercises offer a starting point, consider working with a therapist trained in CBT for personalized guidance and support.

Practice Makes Progress: CBT is a skill that needs regular practice. Diligently engage in the exercises and thought-challenging techniques to see a shift in your thinking patterns.

Be Patient and Kind to Yourself: Changing thought patterns takes time and effort. Don't get discouraged if you don't see immediate results. Celebrate small victories and acknowledge your progress.

The Untold Truth: Empowering Yourself

CBT equips you with powerful tools to challenge negative thought patterns, manage stress and anxiety, and ultimately protect your heart. Remember, you're not powerless against these challenges. By actively engaging in CBT exercises and cultivating a growth mindset, you can rewrite the narrative and empower yourself to create a calmer, more heart-healthy life. Embrace the journey of self-discovery, and witness the positive impact it has on your well-being.

CHAPTER SIX

BUILDING RESILIENCE: THE POWER OF OPTIMISM AND SOCIAL CONNECTION

"The greatest obstacle to discovery is not ignorance - it is the illusion of knowledge," declared Daniel J. Boorstin. This profound quote resonates deeply when considering the battle against heart disease. For too long, the focus has been solely on traditional risk factors like cholesterol and blood pressure. However, the untold truth lies in the power of our own minds and the social connections that nourish us. This chapter explores the vital role of optimism and social connection in building resilience against chronic stress and ultimately safeguarding your heart health.

The Optimism Advantage: Seeing the Glass Half Full

Optimism is often dismissed as a naive outlook on life. However, research paints a different picture. Optimists tend to have a more positive outlook on challenges, view setbacks as temporary roadblocks, and believe in their ability to overcome obstacles. This positive mindset translates into significant benefits for heart health:

Stress Buffer: Optimists tend to experience lower stress levels in response to challenges. This reduces the wear and tear on the cardiovascular system caused by chronic stress hormones.

Enhanced Health Behaviors: Optimists are more likely to engage in healthy behaviors like regular exercise and a balanced diet, further reducing their risk of heart disease.

Stronger Immune System: Studies suggest that optimism may bolster the immune system, strengthening the body's defense mechanisms against various health concerns.

The Power of "Yet": Adding a Growth Mindset to Optimism

Optimism is a powerful tool, but it's not about blind positivity. Combining optimism with a growth mindset, the belief that you can learn and improve through effort, creates a potent force. This growth mindset allows you to reframe challenges as opportunities for learning and growth. Instead of viewing setbacks as failures, you view them as a chance to say, "I haven't mastered this yet," fostering resilience and a more optimistic outlook.

Cultivating Optimism: It's a Skill You Can Develop

While some individuals naturally gravitate towards optimism, it's a skill that can be cultivated. Here are some strategies to embrace a more optimistic outlook:

Focus on the Positive: Train your brain to seek out the positive aspects of your life, big or small. Express gratitude for the good things that happen and savor positive experiences.

Challenge Negative Thoughts: Don't let negative self-talk go unchecked. Learn to identify and challenge self-defeating thoughts, replacing them with more realistic and empowering affirmations.

Visualize Success: Spend time visualizing yourself achieving your goals or overcoming challenges. This mental rehearsal can boost your confidence and optimism.

Focus on the Effort, Not Just the Outcome: Celebrate your effort and progress, even if you don't achieve the desired outcome immediately. Focusing on the journey fosters a growth mindset and fosters optimism.

The Strength of Social Connection: You Are Not Alone

Humans are social creatures, and the quality of our social connections profoundly impacts our well-being. Strong social connections provide a sense of belonging, support, and love, acting as a buffer against stress and anxiety. Here's how social connection protects your heart health:

Reduced Stress Response: Social support can help regulate the stress response and lower stress hormone levels, protecting your cardiovascular system.

Enhanced Emotional Regulation: Feeling connected to others can provide a sense of security and promote more balanced emotional responses to challenges.

Increased Physical Activity: Social connections can motivate you to engage in activities with others, leading to increased physical activity and improved cardiovascular health.

Building a Strong Social Network: Fostering Connections

While social media has its place, real-life connections are irreplaceable. Here are some ways to nurture a strong social network:

Invest in Existing Relationships: Make time for your loved ones – friends, family, and romantic partners. Nurture your existing connections through regular communication and spending quality time together.

Seek Out New Connections: Join clubs, volunteer in your community, or take a class to meet new people who share your interests.

Strengthen Weak Ties: Don't underestimate the power of casual connections. Reconnect with old friends, build rapport with your neighbors, or strike up conversations with people you meet in your daily life.

Social Connection: Beyond the Numbers

The benefits of social connection extend far beyond statistics. It's about feeling seen, heard, and valued. It's about having a shoulder to cry on during challenging times and someone to celebrate victories with. By fostering strong social connections, you create a safety net that supports you through life's ups and downs, ultimately promoting well-being and safeguarding your heart health.

The Untold Truth: It's All Connected

Chronic stress, fueled by negative thought patterns and social isolation, wreaks havoc on your heart health. However, the power lies within you. By cultivating optimism, embracing a growth mindset, and nurturing strong social connections, you build remarkable resilience against stress and anxiety. This inner strength empowers you to navigate challenges with a more positive outlook, fostering a healthier and more fulfilling life.

The Ripple Effect: Building a Heart-Healthy Community

The benefits of optimism and social connection extend beyond the individual. As you cultivate these qualities within yourself, you create a ripple effect, impacting those around you. When you approach life with optimism and offer support to others, you contribute to a more positive and supportive environment for everyone. This fosters a sense of community, further promoting resilience and well-being for all.

Embrace the Journey: A Heart-Healthy Life Awaits

Building resilience against stress and anxiety is an ongoing journey. There will be setbacks and challenges along the way. The key is to embrace the journey, celebrate your progress, and never give up on yourself. Remember, you are not alone in this quest. By incorporating the strategies outlined in this chapter and harnessing the power of optimism and social connection, you empower yourself to create a heart-healthy and fulfilling life.

6.1 The Positive Mindset Advantage: How Optimism Boosts Heart Health Outcomes

For decades, the conversation around heart disease has focused on traditional risk factors like cholesterol and blood pressure. However, the untold truth lies within the realm of our own minds. This subchapter sifts into the compelling research on optimism and its profound impact on heart health. We'll also meet inspiring individuals who, armed with a positive outlook, defied the odds and emerged victorious in their battles for a healthy heart.

Optimism: More Than Just a Sunny Disposition

Optimism is often dismissed as mere cheerfulness, a Pollyannaish outlook on life. But scientific research paints a different picture. Optimists tend to hold a more positive view of challenges, viewing setbacks as temporary hurdles and believing in their capacity to overcome obstacles. This positive mindset translates into significant benefits for heart health:

Stress Buffer: Studies have shown that optimists experience lower stress levels in response to challenges. This translates to a reduced wear and tear on the cardiovascular system caused by chronic stress hormones like cortisol.

Improved Health Behaviors: Optimistic individuals are more likely to embrace healthy behaviors like regular exercise and a balanced diet, further reducing their risk of heart disease.

Enhanced Immune System: Emerging research suggests that optimism may bolster the immune system, strengthening the body's defense mechanisms against various health concerns.

The Science Behind Optimism's Heart-Protective Effects

Let's sift deeper into the science behind optimism's influence on heart health. Here are some key mechanisms:

Neurohormonal Effects: Optimism promotes the release of beneficial neurotransmitters like dopamine and serotonin. These neurotransmitters can lower blood pressure and heart rate, contributing to a healthier cardiovascular system.

Reduced Inflammation: Chronic stress is linked to increased inflammation, a risk factor for heart disease. Optimism can help regulate inflammatory responses, offering a protective effect.

Enhanced Self-Care: A positive outlook can motivate individuals to prioritize self-care behaviors like healthy eating, regular exercise, and preventive healthcare, all crucial for heart health.

The Optimism Advantage in Action: Research Reveals a Clear Connection

Numerous studies have established a clear link between optimism and heart health. Here are some compelling findings:

A major study published in the Journal of the American Medical Association (JAMA) found that optimists had a 35% lower risk of heart attack, stroke, or death from cardiovascular causes compared to their less optimistic counterparts.

Research published in Circulation: Cardiovascular Quality and Outcomes found that optimistic coronary artery disease (CAD) patients were more likely to adhere to their medication regimens and lifestyle changes, leading to improved outcomes.

A study in Psychosomatic Medicine demonstrated that optimists recovering from cardiac events like bypass surgery experienced faster recovery times, highlighting the impact of optimism on overall well-being.

From Skepticism to Strength: Inspiring Stories of Optimism in Action

The power of optimism isn't just a scientific concept; it's exemplified by countless individuals who have overcome immense challenges with a positive mindset. Here are two inspiring stories:

David's Determined Heart: David, a successful businessman, was diagnosed with a life-threatening heart condition at a young age. Initially overwhelmed, he could have easily succumbed to despair. However, David chose a different path. He embraced an optimistic outlook, focusing on the things he could control – his diet, exercise routine, and stress management techniques. He actively participated in his treatment plan, remaining positive and motivated throughout his recovery. Today, David leads a vibrant and active life, a testament to the power of optimism in the face of adversity.

Chelly's Second Chance: Sarah, a mother of two young children, suffered a major heart attack. The fear of leaving her family behind was crippling. Yet, Chelly chose to focus on hope. She visualized herself returning to her children, playing with them, and creating lasting memories. She actively participated in cardiac rehabilitation, fueled by a positive outlook and a determination to regain her health. Chelly's optimism not only aided her recovery but also inspired her family to embrace a healthier lifestyle, creating a ripple effect of positive change.

Beyond Inspiration: Cultivating Optimism in Your Own Life

The stories of David and Chelly showcase the transformative power of optimism. While some individuals naturally gravitate towards a positive outlook, it's a skill that can be cultivated. Here are some strategies to embrace a more optimistic mindset:

- Focus on the Positive: Train your brain to seek out the good in your life, no matter how small. Express gratitude for the blessings you have and savor positive experiences.

- Challenge Negative Thoughts: Don't let negative self-talk go unchecked. Learn to identify and challenge self-defeating thoughts, replacing them with more realistic and empowering affirmations.

- Visualize Success: Spend time visualizing yourself achieving your goals or overcoming challenges. This mental rehearsal can boost your confidence and optimism.

- Focus on the Effort, Not Just the Outcome: Celebrate your effort and progress, even if you don't achieve the desired outcome immediately. Focusing on the journey fosters a growth mindset and fosters optimism.

- Surround Yourself with Positive People: The people you spend time with significantly influence your outlook. Seek out positive and supportive individuals who uplift and inspire you.

- Practice Gratitude: Gratitude is a powerful antidote to negativity. Expressing gratitude for the good things in your life, big or small, shifts your focus towards the positive and fosters optimism.

The Untold Truth: You Hold the Power

The research is clear: optimism is a potent weapon in your fight for a healthy heart. By cultivating a positive outlook and embracing a growth mindset, you empower yourself to manage stress more effectively, prioritize self-care behaviors, and ultimately safeguard your heart health. Remember, the power to create a healthier, more fulfilling life lies within you. Embrace the journey, cultivate optimism, and witness the positive impact it has on your well-being. The choice is yours.

6.2 The Strength of Community: Building Social Support for Well-being

For too long, the conversation surrounding heart health has focused on individual risk factors. However, the untold truth lies in the power of our social connections. Humans are social creatures, and the quality of our relationships profoundly impacts our emotional well-being and, consequently, our heart health. This subchapter explores the importance of social connection, offering strategies for building strong social networks and fostering a sense of belonging, ultimately safeguarding your heart.

The Strength of Social Connection: You Are Not Alone

Social connections provide a sense of belonging, support, and love. They act as a buffer against stress and anxiety, offering a safe space to share burdens, celebrate victories, and receive encouragement. Here's how strong social networks contribute to a healthy heart:

Reduced Stress Response: Social support can help regulate the stress response and lower stress hormone levels, protecting your cardiovascular system. Sharing challenges with loved ones allows you to process emotions in a healthy way, reducing the strain on your heart.

Enhanced Emotional Regulation: Feeling connected to others can provide a sense of security and promote more balanced emotional responses to challenges. Knowing you have a support system can lessen the feeling of being overwhelmed, fostering emotional well-being.

Increased Physical Activity: Social connections can motivate you to engage in activities with others, leading to increased physical activity and improved cardiovascular health. Whether it's a brisk walk with a friend or participating in a group fitness class, social interaction encourages movement, benefiting your heart.

Beyond the Numbers: The Emotional Significance of Connection

The benefits of social connection extend far beyond statistics. It's about feeling seen, heard, and valued. It's about having a shoulder to cry on during challenging times and someone to celebrate victories with. Strong social connections provide a sense of purpose and belonging, fostering a sense of self-worth that contributes to overall well-being.

The Social Connection Deficiency: A Modern Epidemic

In today's fast-paced world, social isolation is a growing concern. The rise of technology, while offering opportunities for connection, can also contribute to feelings of loneliness and isolation. This lack of social connection can have a significant negative impact on our hearts.

Weaving a Stronger Social Tapestry: Strategies for Building Connection

Building and maintaining strong social connections requires effort but the rewards are immeasurable. Here are some strategies to foster a sense of belonging and cultivate a strong social network:

Invest in Existing Relationships: Nurture your existing connections with friends, family, and romantic partners. Make time for regular communication and prioritize quality time together. Plan activities, share meals, and simply be present for one another.

Seek Out New Connections: Step outside your comfort zone and explore new ways to meet people. Join clubs, volunteer in your community, or take a class to connect with individuals who share your interests. Strike up conversations with people you meet in your daily life – at the grocery store, coffee shop, or dog park.

Strengthen Weak Ties: Don't underestimate the power of casual connections. Reconnect with old friends, build rapport with your neighbors, or chat with the barista at your favorite coffee shop. These seemingly small interactions can create a sense of belonging and expand your social network.

Embrace Your Vulnerability: The Power of Authenticity

Building strong social connections requires authenticity. Let go of the need to portray a perfect image and embrace your vulnerabilities. People connect with genuine individuals who share their struggles and triumphs. Being open and honest allows others to connect with you on a deeper level, fostering stronger relationships.

Fostering a Sense of Belonging: It's a Two-Way Street

Building strong social connections isn't just about acquiring more friends or acquaintances. It's about being a good friend, partner, and family member yourself. Be present for others, offer support, and actively listen. Show genuine interest in the lives of those around you and celebrate their successes. By nurturing reciprocity in your relationships, you contribute to a web of strong connections that benefit everyone.

The Untold Truth: You Are the Architect of Your Social Life

The quality of your social connections significantly impacts your emotional well-being and your heart health. The good news is that you have the power to create a vibrant social tapestry. By implementing the strategies outlined in this chapter and embracing the power of social connection, you can foster a sense of belonging, build a network of support, and ultimately create a healthier and happier life. Remember, you are not meant to navigate life

alone. Reach out, connect with others, and experience the
joy and protection that strong social connections offer.

CHAPTER SEVEN

THE FOOD REVOLUTION: BUILDING A HEART-HEALTHY DIET

"Let food be thy medicine and medicine be thy food," advised Hippocrates, the father of medicine.

This ancient wisdom resonates deeply in the battle against heart disease. For far too long, the focus has been on pharmaceutical interventions and procedures, neglecting the power we hold on our plates. The untold truth lies in the food revolution – a conscious shift towards a heart-healthy diet that empowers you to take control of your health and safeguard your heart.

The Standard American Diet: A Recipe for Disaster

The typical Western diet, brimming with processed foods, saturated fats, added sugars, and refined carbohydrates, creates a perfect storm for heart disease. These foods contribute to:

Elevated Cholesterol Levels: Excessive saturated and trans fats clog arteries, hindering blood flow and increasing the risk of heart attack and stroke.

Increased Blood Pressure: High sodium intake, a hallmark of processed foods, can elevate blood pressure, putting additional strain on your heart.

Chronic Inflammation: Processed foods and refined sugars trigger inflammatory responses in the body, contributing to the development of heart disease.

The Food Revolution: A Paradigm Shift

The food revolution is not about fad diets or deprivation. It's about embracing a sustainable, whole-foods-based approach that nourishes your body and empowers you to make informed choices for a healthy heart. Here are the core principles of this revolution:

Prioritize Whole Foods: Fill your plate with unprocessed, nutrient-dense whole foods like fruits, vegetables, whole grains, legumes, nuts, and seeds. These foods offer a wealth of vitamins, minerals, fiber, and antioxidants, all crucial for cardiovascular health.

Embrace Plant-Based Power: Studies consistently show the benefits of plant-based diets for heart health. Focus on incorporating a variety of fruits, vegetables, legumes, and whole grains while strategically limiting animal products, especially red meat and processed meats.

Healthy Fats are Your Friends: Not all fats are created equal. Prioritize healthy fats like those found in olive oil, avocado, nuts, and seeds. These fats improve cholesterol profiles, reduce inflammation, and contribute to a sense of satiety.

Limit Added Sugars and Refined Carbs: Excessive intake of added sugars and refined carbohydrates can wreak havoc on your blood sugar levels and contribute to weight gain, both risk factors for heart disease. Limit sugary drinks, processed pastries, and refined grains like white bread and white rice.

Mindful Eating: Slow down, savor your food, and pay attention to your body's hunger and fullness cues. Mindful eating promotes healthy portion control and prevents overeating, a factor that can contribute to heart disease.

Building a Heart-Healthy Plate: A Culinary Adventure

Embracing the food revolution doesn't have to be bland or restrictive. There's a world of delicious, heart-healthy options waiting to be explored. Here are some tips to build a vibrant and satisfying plate:

Become a Rainbow Eater: Fill your plate with a variety of colorful fruits and vegetables. Each color represents a unique set of health-promoting nutrients.

Spice Up Your Life: Explore the world of herbs and spices to add flavor to your meals without relying on salt or unhealthy fats.

Get Creative with Whole Grains: Go beyond white rice and pasta. Explore options like quinoa, brown rice, oats, and barley for added fiber and nutrients.

Beans are a Heart-Healthy Powerhouse: Incorporate a variety of beans and lentils into your diet. These legumes are packed with protein, fiber, and heart-healthy nutrients.

Don't Fear Healthy Fats: Drizzle your salad with olive oil, sprinkle your dishes with nuts and seeds, or enjoy a slice of avocado toast. Healthy fats add flavor and satiety to your meals.

Beyond the Plate: Making the Food Revolution a Lifestyle

The food revolution is more than just changing what you eat. It's about cultivating a holistic approach to food and health. Here are some additional strategies to embrace this lifestyle:

Read Food Labels: Become an informed consumer by understanding food labels. Pay attention to serving sizes, saturated and trans-fat content, added sugars, and sodium levels.

Plan Your Meals: Plan your meals and snacks for the week to avoid unhealthy choices when hunger strikes. This helps you stay on track with your heart-healthy goals.

Cook More at Home: Cooking at home allows you to control the ingredients and portion sizes of your meals. Experiment with new recipes and discover the joy of creating delicious and nutritious dishes.

Support Local Farmers Markets: Purchasing fresh produce from local farmers' markets not only ensures quality and taste but also supports your local community.

The Untold Truth: You Are the Chef of Your Health

The food revolution empowers you to take control of your health through conscious dietary choices. By embracing a whole-foods-based approach, prioritizing plant-based power, and strategically incorporating healthy fats, you can create delicious and nutritious meals that nourish your body and safeguard your heart.

The Power of Community: Sharing Your Culinary Journey

The food revolution is more fulfilling when shared. Cook meals with loved ones, explore new recipes together, and celebrate your commitment to healthy eating. Join online communities or cooking classes focused on heart-healthy food. Sharing your culinary journey with others fosters support, accountability, and a sense of belonging, making the transition to a healthy lifestyle more enjoyable.

Beyond Heart Health: The Ripple Effect of Healthy Eating

The benefits of the food revolution extend far beyond your heart. A diet rich in whole foods, fruits, and vegetables provides your body with the nutrients it needs to function optimally, boosting your energy levels, promoting cognitive function, and strengthening your immune system.

The Untold Truth: It's a Delicious Journey

The food revolution is not about deprivation or bland meals. It's about discovering a world of vibrant, flavorful, and heart-healthy dishes. It's about empowering yourself to make informed choices, nourish your body, and safeguard your well-being. Embrace the journey, experiment with new flavors, and celebrate the positive impact of healthy eating on your heart and your overall health. Remember, you are the chef of your health – create a culinary masterpiece that nourishes your body and delights your taste buds.

7.1 Beyond Fads: Understanding the Science of Nutrition for Heart Health

The quest for a healthy heart can be riddled with confusing information. Fad diets and conflicting advice abound, leaving you wondering what to believe. This subchapter sifts into common dietary myths and fads, debunking them with scientific evidence. We'll then explore the science-backed principles of a heart-healthy eating plan, empowering you to make informed choices for your well-being.

The Myth of the Perfect Diet: One Size Doesn't Fit All

The internet and media are saturated with claims of "miracle" diets promising rapid weight loss and improved heart health. The truth is, there's no single "perfect" diet for everyone. Individual needs, preferences, and health conditions play a significant role. Focus on a sustainable, flexible approach that fits your lifestyle and allows for long-term adherence.

Myth Busters: Debunking Common Dietary Fads

Let's debunk some of the most pervasive dietary myths:

Myth #1: Fat is Evil: Not all fats are created equal. Saturated and trans fats found in processed foods and red meat contribute to heart disease. However, healthy fats like those found in olive oil, avocado, nuts, and seeds offer numerous benefits for heart health. Include these healthy fats in moderation as part of a balanced diet.

Myth #2: Carbs are the Enemy: Just like fats, there are good and bad carbs. Refined carbohydrates like white bread, white rice, and sugary drinks spike blood sugar levels and increase your risk of heart disease. However, complex carbohydrates like whole grains, fruits, and vegetables provide essential fiber, vitamins, and minerals, promoting satiety and supporting heart health.

Myth #3: All Calories Are Created Equal: While calorie intake plays a role in weight management, it doesn't tell the whole story. The quality of the calories you consume matters. A calorie from a sugary donut has a different impact on your body compared to a calorie from a nutrient-dense avocado. Focus on whole, unprocessed foods to fuel your body with essential nutrients.

Myth #4: Detox Diets are the Answer: Our bodies have built-in detoxification systems like the liver and kidneys. Extreme detox diets can be restrictive, deprive your body of essential nutrients, and even be harmful. Focus on a balanced diet rich in fruits, vegetables, and whole grains to support your body's natural detoxification process.

Beyond the Fads: The Science Behind a Heart-Healthy Diet

While there's no one-size-fits-all approach, several science-backed principles form the foundation of a heart-healthy eating plan:

Prioritize Plant-Based Power: Numerous studies have shown the significant benefits of plant-based diets for heart health. Aim to fill your plate with fruits, vegetables, whole grains, legumes, and nuts. These foods are packed with fiber, antioxidants, and essential nutrients that protect your heart.

Limit Added Sugars and Refined Carbs: Excessive intake of added sugars and refined carbohydrates can contribute to weight gain, elevated blood sugar levels, and increased risk of heart disease. Replace sugary drinks with water or unsweetened tea, and opt for whole grains like brown rice or quinoa instead of white bread or pasta.

Choose Healthy Fats Wisely: Healthy fats like those found in olive oil, avocado, nuts, and seeds are essential for heart health. They improve cholesterol profiles, reduce inflammation, and contribute to a sense of satiety. Incorporate these fats into your diet in moderation.

Focus on Whole, Unprocessed Foods: The foundation of a heart-healthy diet lies in whole, unprocessed foods. These foods are naturally nutrient-rich and provide your body with the building blocks it needs for optimal function. Limit processed foods that are often high in unhealthy fats, added sugars, and sodium.

Mindful Eating Practices: Pay attention to your body's hunger and fullness cues. Eat slowly, savor your food, and avoid distractions while eating. Mindful eating promotes healthy portion control and prevents overeating, a factor that can contribute to heart disease.

The Untold Truth: Sustainability is Key

The key to a heart-healthy diet lies not in quick fixes or restrictive fads, but in a sustainable approach you can maintain long-term. Experiment with different recipes, discover new flavors, and find healthy options you enjoy.

This will help you stay on track and reap the long-term benefits of a heart-healthy diet.

Building Your Heart-Healthy Plate: A Recipe for Success

Here are some practical tips to build a heart-healthy plate:

- Fill Half Your Plate with Colorful Produce: Aim for a variety of colorful fruits and vegetables at every meal. Each color represents a unique set of health-promoting nutrients.

- Choose Whole Grains Over Refined Options: Swap white bread, pasta, and rice for whole-grain alternatives like brown rice, quinoa, whole-wheat bread, and oats. These offer more fiber, vitamins, and minerals, promoting satiety and supporting heart health.

- Incorporate Healthy Fats Wisely: Drizzle your salad with olive oil, add a handful of nuts or seeds to your yogurt, or enjoy a slice of avocado toast. Healthy fats add flavor and satiety to your meals while supporting your heart.

- Embrace Plant-Based Protein Power: Beans, lentils, and peas are excellent sources of protein and fiber, making them perfect additions to a heart-healthy diet. Explore vegetarian chili, lentil soup, or bean salads to incorporate these versatile plant-based proteins.

- Limit Red Meat and Processed Meats: Red meat consumption should be limited, and processed meats like bacon, sausage, and deli meats should be minimized due to their high saturated fat and sodium content. opt for lean protein sources like fish, poultry, or plant-based alternatives when possible.

Season with Flavor, Not Salt: Sodium is a major concern for heart health. Limit processed foods that are often high in sodium. Experiment with herbs, spices, and citrus to add flavor to your meals naturally.

The Power of Small Changes: Building Momentum for a Heart-Healthy Lifestyle

Making significant dietary changes all at once can be overwhelming. Focus on small, sustainable changes you can incorporate into your routine. Here are some ideas:

Start with One Meal a Day: Begin by making your breakfast, lunch, or dinner heart-healthy. Gradually incorporate healthy choices into your other meals.

Swap Sugary Drinks for Water: Replace sugary drinks like soda, juice, and sports drinks with water, unsweetened tea, or black coffee. This simple change significantly reduces your sugar intake and promotes heart health.

Snack Smarter: Choose nutrient-dense snacks like fruits, vegetables with hummus, nuts, or yogurt. Avoid processed snacks that are often high in unhealthy fats, added sugars, and sodium.

Cook More at Home: Cooking at home allows you to control the ingredients and portion sizes of your meals.

Experiment with new recipes and discover the joy of creating delicious and nutritious dishes.

Celebrate Your Successes: Acknowledge your progress, no matter how small. Celebrate your commitment to a heart-healthy lifestyle and reward yourself with non-food related incentives.

The Untold Truth: You Are the Architect of Your Plate

By debunking dietary myths and focusing on the science-backed principles of a heart-healthy eating plan, you empower yourself to make informed choices about your well-being. Embrace a sustainable approach, prioritize whole foods, and gradually incorporate changes that fit your lifestyle. Remember, small changes can lead to significant results. Become the architect of your plate and create a delicious and nutritious foundation for a healthy heart and a fulfilling life.

7.2 Creating a Sustainable Eating Plan: Delicious and Nutritious Choices

Eating for heart health doesn't have to be bland or restrictive. It's about embarking on a delicious culinary adventure, filled with vibrant flavors and satisfying meals. This subchapter equips you with practical meal planning tips and heart-healthy recipe suggestions, empowering you to transform your kitchen into a haven of nutritious and enjoyable meals.

Planning for Success: Building a Heart-Healthy Meal Plan

Meal planning is a valuable tool for creating a heart-healthy diet. It saves time, reduces stress, and ensures you have healthy options readily available. Here are some tips to get you started:

Schedule Your Planning Sessions: Dedicate time each week to plan your meals and snacks. This helps you stay organized and avoid unhealthy last-minute choices.

Take Inventory: Check your pantry, refrigerator, and freezer to see what ingredients you already have on hand. Plan your meals around these existing ingredients to reduce food waste and save money.

Consider Dietary Needs and Preferences: Do you have any allergies or dietary restrictions? Consider these factors when planning your meals and cater to individual preferences within your household.

Variety is Key: Incorporate a diverse range of fruits, vegetables, whole grains, and lean protein sources throughout the week to ensure you're getting a variety of essential nutrients.

Embrace Batch Cooking: Consider preparing large batches of soup, chili, or stew on the weekend that can be portioned and enjoyed throughout the week. This saves time during busy days and ensures you have healthy options readily available.

Utilize Leftovers Creatively: Leftovers can be a goldmine for creative meals. Transform leftover grilled chicken into a salad, or use leftover roasted vegetables in an omelette.

From Fridge to Flavor: Sample Heart-Healthy Meal Ideas

Now, let's translate these planning tips into delicious reality. Here are some sample meal ideas for breakfast, lunch, dinner, and snacks, showcasing how to prioritize heart-healthy ingredients while tantalizing your taste buds:

Heart-Healthy Breakfast Options:

- Overnight Oats: This fiber-rich and protein-packed breakfast is perfect for busy mornings. Combine rolled oats with your favorite milk (dairy or plant-based), chia seeds, chopped nuts, and sliced fruit. Refrigerate overnight and enjoy a cool, refreshing breakfast in the morning.

- Scrambled Eggs with Smoked Salmon and Whole-Wheat Toast: Eggs are a fantastic source of protein, while smoked salmon adds a healthy dose of omega-3 fatty acids. Serve with whole-wheat toast for added fiber and a satisfying start to your day.

- Greek Yogurt with Berries and Granola: This protein and fiber-rich combination is a delicious and nutritious breakfast option. opt for plain Greek yogurt and top it with fresh berries and a sprinkle of heart-healthy granola.

Lunchtime Delights for a Healthy Heart:

- Mediterranean Chickpea Salad Sandwich: This vegetarian option is packed with protein and fiber. Combine cooked chickpeas with chopped vegetables like tomato, cucumber, red onion, and Kalamata olives. Dress with a lemon-tahini sauce and serve on whole-wheat bread.

- Salmon Salad with Quinoa: Grilled salmon is a fantastic source of lean protein and healthy fats. Pair it with a bed of quinoa, cooked vegetables like broccoli or asparagus, and a light vinaigrette dressing for a satisfying and nutritious lunch.

- Lentil Soup with Whole-Wheat Bread: This hearty and flavorful soup is a perfect winter lunch option. Lentils are a great source of plant-based protein and fiber, while vegetables add essential vitamins and minerals. Enjoy it with a slice of whole-wheat bread for dipping.

Dinnertime Delectable Heart-Healthy Options:

- Baked Salmon with Roasted Vegetables: Salmon is a heart-healthy superstar with its omega-3 fatty acids. Season salmon with your favorite herbs and spices, then bake it in the oven with a variety of colorful roasted vegetables like Brussels sprouts, broccoli, and sweet potatoes.

- Turkey Chili: This flavorful chili is a perfect one-pot meal packed with protein and fiber. Ground turkey provides lean protein, while kidney beans, black beans, and corn add fiber and essential nutrients. Enjoy with a dollop of plain Greek yogurt or sour cream and a sprinkle of avocado for a complete and satisfying meal.

- Whole-Wheat Pasta with Lentil Bolognese Sauce: Swap traditional red meat for lentils in your bolognese sauce. Lentils provide a plant-based protein source, and the sauce can be simmered with vegetables like carrots, celery, and onions for added flavor and nutrition. Serve over whole-wheat pasta for a satisfying and healthy comfort food option.

Heart-Healthy Snacking: Fueling Your Day with Flavor

Snacking strategically can help you manage hunger and maintain healthy blood sugar levels. Here are some heart-healthy snack ideas:

- . Fruit and Nut Pairing: Pair a piece of fresh fruit like an apple, pear, or banana with a handful of almonds, walnuts, or cashews. This combination provides a satisfying mix of fiber, healthy fats, and natural sweetness.

- Veggies with Hummus: Cut-up vegetables like carrots, bell peppers, celery, or cucumber sticks are a refreshing and crunchy snack. Pair them with a serving of hummus, a delicious dip made from chickpeas, tahini, olive oil, and lemon juice. Hummus offers protein and healthy fats, making this a well-balanced snack.

- Greek Yogurt with Berries: Greek yogurt is a fantastic source of protein and calcium. Opt for plain Greek yogurt and top it with a variety of fresh berries for a delicious and nutritious snack. This option also provides a good dose of antioxidants.

- Hard-Boiled Eggs: Hard-boiled eggs are a convenient and portable protein-rich snack. They are a great source of choline, essential for brain health, and also offer healthy fats and vitamins.

- Trail Mix (DIY Version): Make your own trail mix to control ingredients and ensure a heart-healthy option. Combine nuts, seeds, dried fruit (without added sugar), and whole-grain cereal for a satisfying mix of protein, fiber, and healthy fats.

- Edamame: Edamame, young soybeans in their pods, are a great source of plant-based protein and fiber. They are readily available frozen, making them a convenient snack option. Simply steam or boil them for a few minutes and enjoy them with a sprinkle of sea salt.

- Roasted Chickpeas: Roasting chickpeas transforms them into a crunchy and flavorful snack. Toss chickpeas with olive oil, your favorite spices (think cumin, paprika, garlic powder), and roast them in the oven until crispy. This satisfying snack provides protein, fiber, and healthy fats.

Beyond the Recipe: Building a Flavorful Heart-Healthy Lifestyle

These are just a few examples to spark your creativity. The possibilities for heart-healthy meals and snacks are endless. Here are some additional tips to keep your culinary journey exciting:

Explore New Spices and Herbs: Experiment with different herbs and spices to add flavor to your dishes without relying on salt. Try turmeric, ginger, chili powder, or smoked paprika for a taste explosion.

Embrace Seasonal Produce: Take advantage of seasonal fruits and vegetables at their peak of freshness and flavor. This not only supports local farmers but also ensures you're getting the most nutrients from your produce.

Get Your Kids Involved: Cooking with your children is a fun and educational experience. Let them help you choose recipes, wash vegetables, and stir ingredients. This fosters a positive connection with healthy food and empowers them to make healthy choices in the future.

Make Healthy Swaps: There are many ways to make heart-healthy swaps in your favorite recipes. Use brown rice instead of white rice, ground turkey instead of ground beef, or whole-wheat tortillas instead of flour tortillas. These small changes can significantly improve the heart-health profile of your meals without sacrificing flavor.

The Untold Truth: You Are the Master Chef of Your Kitchen

By following these tips and incorporating heart-healthy ingredients into your meals and snacks, you transform your kitchen into a haven of delicious and nutritious creations. Remember, healthy eating doesn't have to be bland or restrictive. Embrace the journey, experiment with new flavors, and discover the joy of creating meals that nourish your heart and tantalize your taste buds. You are the master chef of your kitchen; create a culinary masterpiece that fuels your well-being and celebrates the vibrant world of heart-healthy food.

CHAPTER EIGHT

MOVE YOUR BODY, MOVE YOUR HEART: THE POWER OF EXERCISE

For decades, the conversation surrounding heart disease has painted a picture of a ticking time bomb – a relentless progression towards an inevitable event. This narrative has instilled fear and a sense of powerlessness. The untold truth about heart disease challenges this paradigm. It empowers you to take control of your heart health, not through passive acceptance, but through active participation.

The Enemy Within: Unveiling the Risk Factors

Heart disease remains the leading cause of death globally. While genetics play a role, numerous modifiable risk factors significantly influence your heart health. Understanding these factors empowers you to make informed choices and implement strategies for a healthier heart.

Unhealthy Diet: A diet brimming with processed foods, saturated fats, added sugars, and refined carbohydrates contributes to heart disease. These foods elevate cholesterol levels, increase blood pressure, and promote inflammation – a recipe for cardiovascular trouble.

Physical Inactivity: A sedentary lifestyle is detrimental to heart health. Regular physical activity strengthens your heart muscle, improves blood flow, and helps maintain a healthy weight, all crucial for reducing your risk of heart disease.

Smoking: Smoking is one of the most significant risk factors for heart disease. The chemicals in cigarettes damage blood vessels, promote inflammation, and increase the risk of blood clots.

Obesity: Excess weight puts a strain on your heart, contributing to high blood pressure, insulin resistance, and sleep apnea, all of which elevate your risk of heart disease.

Stress: Chronic stress wreaks havoc on your cardiovascular system. It releases stress hormones that increase blood pressure and heart rate, and can also lead to unhealthy coping mechanisms like overeating or smoking.

Diabetes: Diabetes significantly increases your risk of heart disease. High blood sugar levels damage blood vessels and contribute to inflammation, creating a perfect storm for cardiovascular complications.

High Blood Pressure and Cholesterol: Uncontrolled high blood pressure and unhealthy cholesterol levels damage blood vessels and arteries, increasing the risk of heart attack and stroke.

Beyond the Numbers: The Emotional Impact of Heart Disease

Heart disease isn't just a physical condition; it significantly impacts your emotional well-being. The fear of a heart attack, the limitations imposed by the disease, and the lifestyle changes required can all lead to anxiety, depression, and social isolation. Addressing the emotional aspects of heart disease is crucial for your overall well-being.

The Untold Truth: You Are Not a Passive Bystander

The good news is that you are not powerless in the face of heart disease. While you can't change your genetics, you can significantly influence your risk factors through lifestyle modifications. Here's how you can take control of your heart health:

Embrace a Heart-Healthy Diet: Fill your plate with whole, unprocessed foods like fruits, vegetables, whole grains, legumes, nuts, and seeds. Limit saturated and trans fats, added sugars, and refined carbohydrates. This dietary shift empowers you to nourish your body with the nutrients it needs to thrive.

Move Your Body: Engage in regular physical activity. Aim for at least 150 minutes of moderate-intensity exercise or 75 minutes of vigorous-intensity exercise per week. Find activities you enjoy, whether it's brisk walking, swimming, cycling, or dancing. Every step count towards a healthier heart.

Manage Stress: Chronic stress is a silent killer. Develop healthy coping mechanisms to manage stress, such as yoga, meditation, deep breathing exercises, or spending time in nature. Prioritize relaxation and activities that bring you joy.

Quit Smoking: If you smoke, quitting is the single most important thing you can do for your heart health. Smoking cessation programs, medication, and support groups can significantly increase your success rate.

Maintain a Healthy Weight: If you're overweight or obese, losing even a moderate amount of weight can significantly improve your heart health. Focus on sustainable lifestyle changes that promote healthy eating and physical activity.

Manage Diabetes and Blood Pressure: If you have diabetes or high blood pressure, working with your doctor to manage these conditions is crucial for protecting your heart. This may involve medication, lifestyle modifications, or a combination of both.

The Power of Prevention: A Proactive Approach to Heart Health

Prevention is always better than cure. Here are some additional strategies for a proactive approach to heart health:

- Get Regular Checkups: Schedule regular checkups with your doctor to monitor your blood pressure, cholesterol levels, and blood sugar. Early detection and intervention are key to preventing heart disease complications.

- Know Your Family History: Understanding your family history of heart disease can help you identify your risk factors and take appropriate preventive measures.

- Get Enough Sleep: Chronic sleep deprivation can contribute to high blood pressure, weight gain, and diabetes, all of which increase your risk of heart disease. Aim for 7-8 hours of quality sleep.

- Befriend Fiber: Fiber plays a vital role in heart health. It helps regulate blood sugar levels, lower cholesterol, and promote a healthy gut microbiome, all contributing to a reduced risk of heart disease. Incorporate plenty of fiber-rich foods into your diet, such as fruits, vegetables, whole grains, legumes, and nuts.

- Discover the Power of Social Connection: Strong social connections are essential for your overall well-being, including your heart health. Social isolation can increase stress and contribute to unhealthy lifestyle choices. Nurture your relationships with loved ones, engage in social activities, and consider joining a support group focused on heart health.

Empowering Others: Sharing Your Heart-Healthy Journey

You are not alone on this journey. Share your experiences and inspire others to prioritize their heart health. Talk to your family and friends about your commitment to healthy living, cook heart-healthy meals together, and encourage each other to make positive changes. By creating a ripple effect, you can empower your loved ones and contribute to a culture of heart health within your community.

The Untold Truth: You Are the Guardian of Your Heart

The power to safeguard your heart lies within you. By making informed choices, embracing a heart-healthy lifestyle, and prioritizing your well-being, you become the guardian of your heart. This is not a passive surrender to fate, but an active commitment to a vibrant and healthy life. The untold truth about heart disease is that you have the power to write a new story, a story of resilience, empowerment, and a heart that beats strong for a lifetime.

8.1 Finding Your Fit: Exercise Options for All Levels and Abilities

Physical activity is a cornerstone of a heart-healthy lifestyle. It strengthens your heart muscle, improves blood flow, and helps maintain a healthy weight – all essential elements in the fight against heart disease. But the thought of exercise can be daunting, especially if you're new to fitness or have limitations. The good news is, there's an exercise option for everyone, regardless of fitness level or ability. Let's delve into a variety of heart-healthy exercises, catering to different needs and preferences.

Finding Your Fitness Fit: Activities for Every Stage

Embrace the Power of Walking: Walking is a simple yet powerful exercise that offers numerous benefits for your heart. It requires minimal equipment, can be done almost anywhere, and is suitable for all fitness levels. Start with short walks and gradually increase the duration and intensity as your fitness improves. Walking briskly for at least 30 minutes most days of the week is a fantastic way to improve your heart health.

The Joy of Swimming: Swimming is a low-impact, full-body exercise that's gentle on your joints. It provides resistance training, improves cardiovascular health, and offers a refreshing way to stay active. Whether you're doing laps or simply enjoying a leisurely swim, you're strengthening your heart and reaping the benefits of this versatile exercise.

Cycling for a Healthy Heart: Cycling is a fun and effective way to get your heart pumping. Whether you hit the open road or cycle indoors on a stationary bike, you're engaging your major muscle groups and giving your cardiovascular system a workout. Cycling is a low-impact option suitable for various fitness levels, allowing you to adjust the intensity based on your needs.

Beyond the Basics: Expanding Your Exercise Horizons

Once you've established a foundation with basic activities like walking, swimming, or cycling, you can explore other avenues for heart-healthy exercise:

Dance Your Way to Fitness: Dust off your dancing shoes! Dancing is a fun and social way to get your heart rate up and improve your coordination. From ballroom dancing to Zumba classes, there's a dance style for everyone. Embrace the rhythm and enjoy the cardiovascular benefits of this joyful activity.

Strength Training for a Stronger Heart: Strength training isn't just about building muscle; it's also beneficial for heart health. Stronger muscles improve your metabolism, help regulate blood sugar levels, and even contribute to better balance, all of which reduce your risk of heart disease. Consider bodyweight exercises, free weights, or resistance bands to incorporate strength training into your routine.

Interval Training for a Boost: Interval training involves alternating periods of high-intensity exercise with periods of rest or low-intensity activity. This dynamic approach elevates your heart rate for short bursts, followed by recovery periods, resulting in a more efficient workout with significant heart-health benefits.

Mind-Body Connection: Exploring Non-Traditional Exercise Options

Exercise doesn't have to be confined to the gym or the outdoors. Here are some alternative options that promote heart health while nurturing a mind-body connection:

Yoga for Heart and Mind: Yoga offers a holistic approach to well-being, combining physical postures (asanas) with breathing exercises (pranayama) and meditation. Yoga improves flexibility, strengthens the core, and promotes relaxation, all contributing to a healthier heart.

Tai Chi for a Gentle Approach: Tai chi is an ancient Chinese practice that combines gentle movements with deep breathing and meditation. This low-impact exercise improves balance, flexibility, and reduces stress, all of which benefit your heart health.

Pilates for Core Strength: Pilates focuses on strengthening your core muscles, which are essential for good posture and stability. Strong core muscles improve your overall fitness and can also contribute to a healthier heart.

Listen to Your Body: Tailoring Exercise to Your Needs

The key to a sustainable exercise routine is finding activities you enjoy and that fit your current fitness level. If you have any limitations or health concerns, it's crucial to consult your doctor before starting a new exercise program. Here are some additional tips for tailoring exercise to your needs:

- Start Slowly and Gradually Increase Intensity: Don't try to do too much too soon. Begin with shorter durations and lower intensity, and gradually increase them as your fitness improves.

- Listen to Your Body: Pay attention to your body's signals. If you experience pain or discomfort, stop the activity and rest.

- Find Activities You Enjoy: Exercise should be enjoyable, not a chore. Explore different activities and find ones you truly love, making it easier to stick with your routine.

- Make it Social: Exercise with a friend, join a fitness class, or find a workout buddy. Social support can make exercise more fun and help you stay accountable. Having someone to share the experience with can provide motivation, encouragement, and even a healthy dose of friendly competition. Consider joining a walking group, a local sports team, or a dance class. The social aspect can make exercise feel less like a chore and more like a fun activity.

- Embrace Technology: There are numerous fitness apps and online resources that can help you track your progress, find new workout routines, and stay motivated. Some apps offer guided workouts, virtual fitness classes, and even personalized training plans. Explore the options and find technology that complements your exercise routine.

- Make it Fun: Inject some fun into your exercise routine. Explore new activities, listen to upbeat music, or reward yourself for reaching your fitness goals. Keeping things interesting will help you stay motivated and prevent boredom.

Beyond Exercise: Embracing a Holistic Approach to Heart Health

While exercise plays a crucial role in heart health, it's just one piece of the puzzle. Here are some additional lifestyle factors to consider for a holistic approach:

Prioritize Quality Sleep: Chronic sleep deprivation can contribute to a variety of health problems, including heart disease. Aim for 7-8 hours of quality sleep each night to allow your body to rest and repair itself.

Manage Stress: Chronic stress wreaks havoc on your cardiovascular system. Develop healthy coping mechanisms for stress management, such as deep breathing exercises, meditation, or spending time in nature.

Maintain a Healthy Weight: If you're overweight or obese, losing even a moderate amount of weight can significantly improve your heart health. Focus on sustainable lifestyle changes that promote healthy eating and physical activity.

Don't Smoke: Smoking is one of the most significant risk factors for heart disease. If you smoke, quitting is the single most important thing you can do for your heart health.

The Untold Truth: Every Step Counts

The road to a healthy heart is paved with consistent effort, not a single monumental leap. Remember, even small changes can make a big difference in the long run. Don't be discouraged if you can't dedicate an hour to exercise every day. Start with shorter bursts of activity and gradually increase your duration and intensity as your fitness improves. Every step you take, every minute you spend moving your body, contributes to a healthier heart and a more vibrant life.

Embrace the Journey, Celebrate Your Victories

Focus on the journey of becoming more active, not just the destination. Celebrate your victories, big and small. Did you walk for 30 minutes today? Great! Did you manage to attend a fitness class for the first time? Fantastic! Acknowledge your progress and reward yourself for your commitment to a healthier you.

The Untold Truth: You Are the Architect of Your Movement

The power to move your body and prioritize your heart health lies within you. You are the architect of your movement. Explore different activities, find what resonates with you, and create an exercise routine that fits your lifestyle and preferences. Remember, consistency is key. By incorporating regular physical activity into your life, you become an active participant in your well-being, taking charge of your heart health and paving the way for a long and vibrant life.

8.2 Consistency is Key: Building an Exercise Routine You Can Maintain

The path to a heart-healthy lifestyle is paved with consistent movement. But let's face it, life can get busy, and motivation can wane. This subchapter equips you with strategies to build a sustainable exercise routine, conquer common barriers, and reignite your fitness fire, empowering you to move your body and nourish your heart for life.

Crafting Your Exercise Blueprint: Building a Sustainable Routine

A sustainable exercise routine isn't a rigid one-size-fits-all program. It's a personalized blueprint that caters to your lifestyle, preferences, and fitness level. Here are some key elements to consider when crafting your routine:

Find Activities You Enjoy: Exercise shouldn't feel like a chore. Explore different activities – from brisk walking and swimming to dancing and hiking. Discover what brings you joy and keeps you engaged. When you enjoy your workouts, you're more likely to stick with them in the long run.

Schedule Your Workouts: Treat exercise like any other important appointment. Schedule your workouts in your planner and commit to them as you would a meeting or a social engagement. This helps prioritize your well-being and ensures you dedicate time for physical activity.

Start Small and Gradually Progress: Don't overwhelm yourself by jumping into a demanding exercise routine. Begin with shorter durations and lower intensity, and gradually increase them as your fitness improves. Consistency is key, so prioritize regular workouts even if they're shorter at first.

Variety is the Spice of Life (and Exercise): To keep things interesting and prevent boredom, incorporate a variety of activities into your routine. Try a new HIIT (High-Intensity Interval Training) class one day, go for a bike ride the next, and explore a yoga session the following day. This keeps your workouts stimulating and prevents plateaus.

Conquering the Mountain: Overcoming Barriers to Exercise

Life throws curveballs, and sometimes those curveballs can derail your exercise routine. Here are some strategies for overcoming common barriers:

Time Constraints: We all have busy schedules, but carving out time for exercise is an investment in your health. Consider shorter, more efficient workouts or break down your exercise into smaller chunks throughout the day. Even a 10-minute walk is better than nothing.

Lack of Motivation: We all experience dips in motivation. Keep your fitness goals visible by writing them down and placing them somewhere you'll see them every day. Find a workout buddy, join a fitness class, or listen to upbeat music to reignite your exercise fire.

Fear of Failure: Don't be afraid to start small and celebrate your progress, no matter how seemingly insignificant. Focus on the journey of becoming more active, not just the destination. Every step count towards a healthier you.

Lack of Knowledge or Support: Feeling lost about where to begin? Talk to your doctor or a certified personal trainer for guidance. There are also numerous online resources and fitness apps that offer workout routines and support.

Staying Lit: Strategies for Long-Term Motivation

Motivation is a flame that needs tending to. Here are some strategies to keep your fitness fire burning brightly:

Set SMART Goals: Set Specific, Measurable, Achievable, Relevant, and Time-bound goals. These goals should be challenging yet attainable, allowing you to track your progress and celebrate milestones. As you achieve your initial goals, set new ones to keep yourself motivated.

Track Your Progress: Seeing your progress is a fantastic motivator. Use a fitness tracker, journal your workouts, or take progress photos. Tracking your achievements allows you to visualize your journey and celebrate your accomplishments.

Reward Yourself: Positive reinforcement goes a long way. Reward yourself for reaching your fitness goals, whether it's a new workout outfit, a massage, or a fun activity you enjoy. This reinforcement helps solidify the positive association with exercise.

Find a Fitness Community: Surround yourself with like-minded individuals who share your passion for health and fitness. Join a workout group, find a running buddy, or connect with online fitness communities. Having a support system can boost motivation and keep you accountable.

The Untold Truth: You Are the Architect of Your Motivation

Ultimately, the power to stay motivated lies within you. Shift your mindset. Don't view exercise as a punishment for what you eat; see it as a celebration of your body and its potential. Focus on how exercise makes you feel – energized, empowered, and invigorated. When you connect with the positive impact of movement on your well-being, motivation becomes an intrinsic force.

Embrace the Journey, Celebrate the Victories

Remember, building a sustainable exercise routine is a journey, not a destination. There will be setbacks, missed workouts, and days when motivation wanes. Don't beat yourself up. Acknowledge these challenges, accept them as part of the process, and recommit to your goals. Every time you lace up your walking shoes, step onto your yoga mat, or hop on your bike, you're making a positive choice for your heart health. Celebrate these victories, big and small. Did you manage a 30-minute walk even though you were feeling tired? Fantastic! Did you dust off your weights and complete a strength training session after a long break? Celebrate! Recognizing and celebrating your progress, no matter how seemingly insignificant, fuels your motivation and keeps you moving forward on your path to a healthier heart.

The Untold Truth: It's a Marathon, not a Sprint

Think of your exercise routine as a marathon, not a sprint. Sustainability is key. Focus on consistency over intensity. It's better to engage in regular, moderate-intensity exercise than to push yourself to the limit only to fizzle out after a few weeks. Gradually increase the intensity and duration of your workouts as your fitness improves. This steady, sustainable approach is more likely to yield long-term results and empower you to make exercise a lifelong habit.

The Untold Truth: You Are in Control

The power to move your body, nourish your heart, and build a sustainable exercise routine lies within you. You are in control. Take charge of your health and well-being. Embrace the joy of movement, celebrate your victories, and trust in your ability to create a lifestyle that keeps your heart healthy and your spirit vibrant. With dedication, consistency, and a commitment to self-care, you can transform exercise from a chore into a celebration of life, empowering you to write a new story – a story of resilience, motivation, and a heart that beats strong for a lifetime.

CHAPTER NINE

SLEEP: THE UNDERRATED PILLAR OF HEART HEALTH

For decades, the conversation surrounding heart disease has painted a picture of clogged arteries, high cholesterol, and the ticking time bomb of a potential heart attack. While these factors undoubtedly play a role, the untold truth about heart health reveals a hidden culprit often relegated to the sidelines – sleep. Chronic sleep deprivation isn't just about daytime fatigue; it's a silent saboteur that significantly increases your risk of heart disease.

Understanding the Science Behind Rest

Sleep is not a passive state of unconsciousness; it's a vital physiological process as crucial to our well-being as a healthy diet or regular exercise. During sleep, our bodies enter a restorative state, repairing tissues, consolidating memories, and regulating hormones. This symphony of biological processes significantly impacts our cardiovascular health.

The Rest and Repair Chorus: Deep sleep triggers the release of growth hormone, essential for cell repair and tissue regeneration. This restorative process strengthens the heart muscle and promotes overall cardiovascular health.

The Hormonal Harmony: Sleep regulates the production of hormones like leptin (promotes satiety) and ghrelin (increases hunger). Chronic sleep deprivation disrupts this hormonal balance, potentially leading to weight gain, a significant risk factor for heart disease.

The Blood Pressure Rhythm: During sleep, blood pressure naturally dips, allowing your heart to rest and recharge. However, chronic sleep deprivation keeps your nervous system in overdrive, contributing to elevated blood pressure and increased strain on your heart.

The Inflammatory Interlude: Sleep plays a crucial role in regulating inflammation, a key player in the development of heart disease. Chronic sleep deprivation disrupts this delicate balance, promoting chronic inflammation and increasing your risk of cardiovascular complications.

The Sleepless: How Chronic Sleep Deprivation Disrupts Heart Health

When we consistently skimp on sleep, this intricate consonance of biological processes goes awry, creating a discord that disrupts heart health in several ways:

Elevated Blood Pressure: Chronic sleep deprivation elevates stress hormones like cortisol, which constrict blood vessels and increase blood pressure, putting a strain on your heart.

Insulin Resistance: Sleep deprivation disrupts the body's ability to regulate blood sugar levels, leading to insulin resistance, a precursor to type 2 diabetes, another significant risk factor for heart disease.

Atherosclerosis Acceleration: Chronic sleep deprivation is linked to increased inflammation and the buildup of plaque in arteries, a condition known as atherosclerosis, which can lead to heart attack and stroke.

Beyond the Numbers: The Ripple Effect of Sleep Deprivation on Heart Health

The consequences of sleep deprivation extend beyond the realm of biological processes. It can also negatively impact your lifestyle choices, further jeopardizing your heart health:

Unhealthy Food Choices: Sleep deprivation disrupts your body's ability to regulate hormones like leptin and ghrelin, leading to increased cravings for unhealthy, high-calorie foods. This can contribute to weight gain and worsen your cardiovascular risk profile.

Physical Inactivity: Chronic fatigue associated with sleep deprivation can make you less motivated to engage in physical activity, another crucial pillar of heart health.

Increased Stress: Sleep deprivation can exacerbate stress, a known trigger for unhealthy coping mechanisms like smoking or overeating, further increasing your risk of heart disease.

The Untold Truth: You Are Not Powerless

The good news is that you're not a passive bystander in the face of sleep deprivation's impact on your heart health. By prioritizing healthy sleep habits, you can become an active participant in protecting your cardiovascular system:

Establish a Regular Sleep Schedule: Go to bed and wake up at consistent times, even on weekends. This helps regulate your body's natural sleep-wake cycle, promoting better quality sleep.

Create a Relaxing Bedtime Routine: Develop a calming bedtime routine that signals to your body it's time to wind down. This could include taking a warm bath, reading a book, or practicing relaxation techniques like deep breathing or meditation.

Optimize Your Sleep Environment: Ensure your bedroom is dark, quiet, and cool. Invest in blackout curtains, earplugs, and a comfortable mattress to create an environment conducive to quality sleep.

Limit Screen Time Before Bed: The blue light emitted from electronic devices like smartphones and laptops can disrupt sleep patterns. Avoid screen time for at least an hour before bed and opt for relaxing activities instead.

Manage Stress: Chronic stress is a significant sleep disruptor. Identify and address the root causes of your stress. Practice relaxation techniques like yoga, meditation, or deep breathing to manage stress and promote better sleep.

Regular Exercise: While vigorous exercise too close to bedtime can interfere with sleep, regular physical activity earlier in the day can actually improve sleep quality.

9.1 The Science of Sleep: How Restfulness Impacts Cardiovascular Function

For decades, the narrative surrounding heart disease has focused on cholesterol, clogged arteries, and the looming threat of a heart attack. While these factors remain crucial, the untold truth about heart health reveals a hidden culprit: sleep deprivation. This subchapter delves into the science of sleep, unveiling its vital role in cardiovascular function and exposing the dangers of chronic sleeplessness.

Beyond Rest: The orchestration of Sleep and Its Impact on the Heart

Sleep isn't merely a period of unconsciousness; it's a complex biological symphony essential for our well-being. During sleep, our bodies enter a restorative state, repairing tissues, consolidating memories, and regulating hormones – all of which significantly impact our cardiovascular health. Here's a closer look at the intricate relationship between sleep and your heart:

The Rest and Repair Chorus: Deep sleep triggers the release of growth hormone, essential for cell repair and tissue regeneration. This restorative process strengthens the heart muscle, promoting better blood flow and overall cardiovascular health.

The Hormonal Harmony: Sleep regulates the production of hormones like leptin (promotes satiety) and ghrelin (increases hunger). Chronic sleep deprivation disrupts this hormonal balance, potentially leading to weight gain, a significant risk factor for heart disease.

The Blood Pressure Rhythm: During sleep, blood pressure naturally dips. This allows your heart to rest and recharge. However, chronic sleep deprivation keeps your nervous system in overdrive, contributing to elevated blood pressure and increased strain on your heart.

The Inflammatory Interlude: Sleep plays a crucial role in regulating inflammation, a key player in the development of heart disease. Chronic sleep deprivation disrupts this delicate balance, promoting chronic low-grade inflammation and increasing your risk of cardiovascular complications.

The Discordant: How Sleep Deprivation Disrupts Heart Health

When we consistently skimp on sleep, this intricate symphony of biological processes goes awry. This creates a discord that disrupts heart health in several ways:

Elevated Blood Pressure: Chronic sleep deprivation elevates stress hormones like cortisol, which constrict blood vessels and increase blood pressure, putting a strain on your heart.

Insulin Resistance: Sleep deprivation disrupts the body's ability to regulate blood sugar levels, leading to insulin resistance. This is a precursor to type 2 diabetes, another significant risk factor for heart disease.

Atherosclerosis Acceleration: Chronic sleep deprivation is linked to increased inflammation and the buildup of plaque in arteries, a condition known as atherosclerosis. This narrowing of arteries can lead to heart attack and stroke.

Beyond the Numbers: The Ripple Effect of Sleep Deprivation on Heart Health

The consequences of sleep deprivation extend beyond the realm of biological processes. It can also negatively impact your lifestyle choices, further jeopardizing your heart health:

Unhealthy Food Choices: Sleep deprivation disrupts your body's ability to regulate hormones like leptin and ghrelin, leading to increased cravings for unhealthy, high-calorie foods. This can contribute to weight gain and worsen your cardiovascular risk profile.

Physical Inactivity: Chronic fatigue associated with sleep deprivation can make you less motivated to engage in physical activity, another crucial pillar of heart health.

Increased Stress: Sleep deprivation can exacerbate stress, a known trigger for unhealthy coping mechanisms like smoking or overeating, further increasing your risk of heart disease.

A Case Study: The Vicious Cycle of Sleep Deprivation and Heart Health

Imagine Ann, a busy professional who consistently prioritizes work over sleep. She averages 5-6 hours of sleep per night, leaving her feeling constantly fatigued. To cope with the exhaustion, she relies on sugary coffee drinks and processed snacks for quick energy boosts. The lack of sleep also disrupts her motivation to exercise, leading to a more sedentary lifestyle. Over time, Ann's chronic sleep deprivation triggers a domino effect:

- Elevated blood pressure due to increased stress hormones
- Increased risk of insulin resistance due to disrupted blood sugar regulation
- Weight gains due to unhealthy food choices and decreased physical activity
- Increased inflammation throughout the body

These factors all contribute to a heightened risk of developing heart disease. Sarah's story exemplifies how sleep deprivation disrupts the delicate balance of cardiovascular health.

The Untold Truth: You Are Not a Passive Bystander

The good news is that you're not powerless in the face of sleep deprivation's impact on your heart health. By prioritizing healthy sleep habits, you can become an active participant in protecting your cardiovascular system:

Establish a Regular Sleep Schedule: Go to bed and wake up at consistent times, even on weekends. This helps regulate your body's natural sleep-wake cycle, promoting better quality sleep.

Create a Relaxing Bedtime Routine: Develop a calming bedtime routine that signals to your body it's time to wind down. This could include taking a warm bath, reading a book in dim light, or practicing relaxation techniques like deep breathing or meditation. Avoid stimulating activities like watching television or working on electronic devices before bed. The blue light emitted from these devices can suppress melatonin production, a hormone essential for sleep regulation.

Optimize Your Sleep Environment: Ensure your bedroom is dark, quiet, and cool. Invest in blackout curtains, earplugs, and a comfortable mattress to create an environment conducive to quality sleep. Consider using a white noise machine to mask any disruptive sounds. A cool room temperature (between 60-67 degrees Fahrenheit) is also optimal for sleep.

Limit Screen Time Before Bed: The blue light emitted from electronic devices like smartphones and laptops can disrupt sleep patterns. Avoid screen time for at least an hour before bed and opt for relaxing activities instead. Consider dimming the lights in your home in the evening to create a more sleep-supportive environment.

Manage Stress: Chronic stress is a significant sleep disruptor. Identify and address the root causes of your stress. Practice relaxation techniques like yoga, meditation, or deep breathing to manage stress and promote better sleep. Regular exercise can also be a powerful tool for stress management, but avoid strenuous workouts too close to bedtime as they can be stimulating.

Regular Exercise: While vigorous exercise too close to bedtime can interfere with sleep, regular physical activity earlier in the day can actually improve sleep quality. Aim for at least 30 minutes of moderate-intensity exercise most days of the week. However, avoid strenuous workouts within 2-3 hours of bedtime.

See a doctor if Needed: If you're struggling with chronic sleep problems despite implementing these strategies, consult a healthcare professional. There may be underlying medical conditions like sleep apnea or insomnia that require treatment. Don't hesitate to seek help; prioritizing healthy sleep is an investment in your overall health and well-being, including your heart.

The Untold Truth: Sleep is a Cornerstone of Heart Health

Sleep is not a luxury; it's a biological necessity. Just as you wouldn't neglect your diet or physical activity, prioritizing quality sleep is essential for a healthy heart. When you prioritize sleep, you're not just giving your body a rest; you're actively protecting your cardiovascular system and promoting long-term well-being. By understanding the science of sleep and its profound impact on heart health, you're empowered to make informed choices and cultivate healthy sleep habits. Remember, a good night's sleep is a vital ingredient in the recipe for a healthy heart. Make sleep a priority, and watch your heart health flourish.

9.2 Creating a Sleep Sanctuary: Strategies for Better Sleep Hygiene

Imagine a space dedicated solely to rejuvenation, a refuge where worries melt away and restorative sleep washes over you. This is your sleep sanctuary – a haven specifically designed to promote quality sleep and bolster your heart health. Here's how to transform your bedroom from a generic space into a sleep-supportive oasis:

Embrace the Darkness: Light disrupts the production of melatonin, a hormone crucial for sleep regulation. Invest in blackout curtains or an eye mask to block out any light pollution from streetlights or electronics. Darkness creates a cave-like environment, signaling to your body that it's time for sleep.

Hush the Noise: External noise can disrupt sleep patterns. Consider earplugs or a white noise machine to mask any disruptive sounds. White noise can be particularly helpful as it provides a constant, soothing background that can drown out intermittent noises.

Temperature Matters: A cool room temperature promotes deeper sleep. Aim for a temperature between 60-67 degrees Fahrenheit. Consider using a thermostat with a sleep mode that automatically adjusts the temperature throughout the night.

Invest in Comfort: Your mattress and pillows are the foundation of a good night's sleep. Ensure your mattress offers adequate support for your body type and is replaced every 7-10 years. Choose pillows that provide proper neck alignment and adjustability for optimal comfort.

Declutter and Depersonalize: A cluttered space can be visually stimulating and create a sense of overwhelm. Declutter your bedroom, removing unnecessary items and leaving only sleep essentials. This creates a calming, minimalist environment conducive to rest.

Embrace the Power of Scents: Certain scents can promote relaxation and improve sleep quality. Consider using lavender essential oil in a diffuser or spraying lavender linen spray on your sheets. Lavender has calming properties that can ease anxiety and promote deeper sleep.

Banish Electronics: The blue light emitted from electronic devices like smartphones and laptops suppresses melatonin production. Avoid using electronics in bed and establish a "tech-free zone" around your sleep sanctuary. Charge your devices outside the bedroom to avoid the temptation of late-night screen time.

Cultivating a Sleep Oasis: Establishing a Healthy Sleep Hygiene Routine

Creating a sleep sanctuary is just one piece of the puzzle. A consistent sleep hygiene routine – a set of practices that promote quality sleep – strengthens the foundation of your sleep fortress. Here are some key practices to incorporate:

Establish a Regular Sleep Schedule: Go to bed and wake up at consistent times, even on weekends. This helps regulate your body's natural sleep-wake cycle, known as your circadian rhythm. Consistency allows your body to anticipate sleep and wakefulness, promoting better sleep quality.

Create a Relaxing Bedtime Routine: Develop a calming pre-sleep ritual that signals to your body it's time to wind down. This could include taking a warm bath, reading a book in dim light, practicing deep breathing exercises, or listening to calming music. Avoid stimulating activities like watching television or working on electronics before bed.

Dim the Lights: Exposure to bright light in the evening can suppress melatonin production. In the hour leading up to bedtime, dim the lights in your home. This creates a more sleep-supportive environment and prepares your body for sleep. Consider using dimmers on your lights or using warm-colored bulbs that emit less blue light.

Power Down Before Bed: Avoid strenuous physical activity within 2-3 hours of bedtime. Exercise can be stimulating and make it harder to fall asleep. However, regular exercise earlier in the day can actually improve sleep quality.

Beware of Naps: While a short nap (20-30 minutes) can be beneficial, long naps or napping too late in the day can disrupt nighttime sleep. If you do choose to nap, keep it short and avoid napping after 3 pm.

Manage Stress: Chronic stress is a major sleep disruptor. Identify your stress triggers and develop healthy coping mechanisms. Practice relaxation techniques like yoga, meditation, or deep breathing to manage stress and promote better sleep.

Create a Sleep-Wake Association: Use your bed primarily for sleep and sex. Avoid working, watching television, or using electronic devices in bed. This creates a strong association between your bed and sleep, making it easier to fall asleep when you get into bed.

Listen to Your Body: If you can't fall asleep after 20 minutes, get out of bed and engage in a relaxing activity in another room until you feel tired. Lying in bed awake can create anxiety and make it harder to fall asleep.

Beyond the Basics: Strategies for Enhancing Sleep Quality

Beyond the core elements of a sleep sanctuary and a healthy sleep hygiene routine, there are additional strategies you can employ to further enhance your sleep quality and fortify your heart health:

Embrace the Power of Sunlight: Exposure to natural sunlight during the day helps regulate your circadian rhythm, making it easier to fall asleep at night. Aim for at least 30 minutes of sunlight exposure in the morning or early afternoon.

Hydration is Key: Dehydration can disrupt sleep patterns. Ensure you're adequately hydrated throughout the day, but avoid excessive fluids close to bedtime to prevent nighttime bathroom trips.

Dietary Choices for a Restful Night: Avoid heavy meals, sugary foods, and caffeine close to bedtime. These can disrupt sleep and make it harder to fall asleep. Opt for a light, healthy dinner a few hours before bed to promote better sleep.

Relaxing Rituals: Incorporate relaxing activities into your bedtime routine. Taking a warm bath, practicing gentle yoga stretches, or listening to calming music can ease your mind and prepare your body for sleep.

Cognitive Behavioral Therapy for Insomnia (CBT-I): If you struggle with chronic sleep problems despite implementing these strategies, consider seeking professional help. CBT-I is a form of therapy that can be highly effective in addressing insomnia and improving sleep quality.

The Untold Truth: Consistency is King (and Queen)

Transforming your bedroom into a sleep sanctuary, establishing a consistent sleep hygiene routine, and exploring additional sleep-enhancing strategies all contribute to a more restful night's sleep. However, the key to unlocking the full benefits lies in consistency. Just like building a strong physical foundation requires regular exercise, a strong sleep foundation requires consistent effort. By faithfully adhering to these practices over time, you'll cultivate a healthy sleep pattern that empowers you to prioritize your heart health and safeguard your long-term well-being.

Remember, Sleep is an investment, not a Luxury

Prioritizing quality sleep isn't a selfish act; it's an investment in your overall health and well-being. When you prioritize sleep, you're not just giving your body a rest; you're actively protecting your heart and laying the groundwork for a vibrant, fulfilling life. Embrace the power of sleep, cultivate your sleep sanctuary, and watch your heart health flourish. By making sleep a priority, you're taking a proactive step towards a healthier, happier you.

CHAPTER TEN

PRECISION MEDICINE: TAILORING TREATMENT TO YOUR UNIQUE RISK

For over a century, the battle against heart disease has been waged on a one-size-fits-all battlefield. Doctors relied on a limited arsenal of treatments, often overlooking the unique biological landscape of each patient. This approach, while effective in some cases, failed to consider the complex interplay of factors that contribute to individual risk. However, a revolutionary force is emerging, poised to transform the way we prevent and treat heart disease – precision medicine.

Beyond Averages: Unveiling the Heterogeneity of Heart Disease

Heart disease, often perceived as a monolithic entity, is far more nuanced. It manifests in a multitude of ways, with varying causes and risk factors. While high cholesterol and high blood pressure remain significant contributors, a patient's genetic makeup, lifestyle habits, and environmental factors all play a crucial role. This heterogeneity, the vast variability in how heart disease presents itself, highlights the limitations of a one-size-fits-all approach.

Precision Medicine: A Personalized Approach to Heart Health

Precision medicine shatters the mold of traditional medicine, ushering in an era of personalized care. It leverages a multi-pronged approach, considering a patient's unique genetic makeup, lifestyle choices, and environmental exposures to create a tailored treatment plan. This shift from a population-based approach to an individualized strategy holds immense promise for revolutionizing heart disease prevention and treatment.

The Power of Personalized Prevention:

Precision medicine empowers doctors to identify individuals at heightened risk for heart disease well before symptoms arise.

Genetic Testing: Advances in genetic testing allow doctors to identify genetic variants that predispose individuals to heart disease. This information allows for early intervention and implementation of preventive measures like lifestyle modifications or targeted medications.

Biomarkers: Analyzing blood or tissue samples for specific biomarkers – biological indicators of disease – can reveal early signs of heart disease progression. This early detection allows for prompt intervention and potentially prevents complications.

Tailoring Treatment to Your Unique Risk Profile:

Precision medicine doesn't stop at prevention; it extends to treatment as well.

Targeted Therapies: By understanding a patient's specific genetic makeup and disease profile, doctors can prescribe medications that are more likely to be effective and have fewer side effects. This personalized approach optimizes treatment outcomes and reduces the risk of adverse reactions.

Lifestyle Modifications: Precision medicine goes beyond medication. Doctors can create personalized lifestyle modification plans based on an individual's risk factors. This could include dietary recommendations, tailored exercise programs, and stress management strategies to address the specific needs of each patient.

A Case Study: Unveiling the Power of Precision Medicine

Imagine John and Diana, both in their 50s with similar cholesterol levels. John has a family history of heart disease, while Diana does not. Through genetic testing, John is found to have a variant that increases his risk of developing heart disease. Based on this information, John's doctor prescribes a low-dose medication alongside a personalized exercise program. Diana, on the other hand, doesn't require medication, but her doctor recommends dietary changes to address her slightly elevated blood pressure. Precision medicine allows for a nuanced approach, tailoring treatment plans to individual risk profiles.

The Untold Truth: Precision Medicine is a journey, not a Destination

Precision medicine is a rapidly evolving field. While significant progress has been made, there's still much to explore. New genetic variants are being discovered, and our understanding of the complex interplay between genes and environment continues to grow. This ongoing exploration necessitates a collaborative effort between researchers, doctors, and patients to move the field forward.

Empowering Patients: Taking Ownership of Your Heart Health

The power of precision medicine extends beyond the realm of doctors and researchers. Patients, empowered with knowledge about their unique risk factors, can become active participants in safeguarding their heart health. This includes:

Understanding Your Family History: Knowing your family history can provide valuable insights into your risk profile.

- Partnering with Your Doctor: Open communication with your doctor allows for a personalized approach to preventive care and treatment.
- Embracing a Healthy Lifestyle: Regardless of your genetic makeup, adopting a healthy lifestyle – including a balanced diet, regular exercise, and stress management – remains crucial for heart health.

The Future of Heart Health: A Personalized Approach for All

Precision medicine offers a beacon of hope in the fight against heart disease. By harnessing the power of personalized risk assessment, targeted therapies, and patient empowerment, we can move towards a future where heart disease prevention and treatment are tailored to the unique needs of each individual. This shift promises not only to improve clinical outcomes but also to empower patients to take charge of their heart health and live longer, healthier lives.

10.1 Genetic Testing: Uncovering Inherited Predispositions

For centuries, the human body remained an enigma, its secrets locked away within the intricate dance of genes. However, in the age of precision medicine, a powerful tool has emerged to illuminate this hidden landscape – genetic testing. This subchapter delves into the world of genetic testing in the context of heart disease, exploring its benefits, limitations, and how it empowers you to take charge of your cardiovascular health.

Beyond Family History: Unveiling the Nuances of Genetic Predisposition

Family history has long been a cornerstone in assessing heart disease risk. Knowing if your parents or siblings have struggled with heart issues provides valuable information. However, family history only paints a partial picture. Genes can be like a complex instruction manual, with variations and mutations influencing our susceptibility to various diseases. Genetic testing offers a deeper level of insight, revealing the unique genetic makeup that contributes to your individual risk of heart disease.

Decoding Your DNA: How Genetic Testing Works

Genetic testing for heart disease typically involves a simple blood test. A small sample of your blood is analyzed to identify specific genes or variations associated with an increased risk of heart disease. These variations, known as polymorphisms, can influence factors like cholesterol levels, blood pressure regulation, and blood clotting. By analyzing your genetic makeup, doctors gain valuable insights into your predisposition to develop heart disease.

Genetic testing for heart disease offers several key benefits:

Early Risk Assessment: Identifying genetic variants associated with heart disease allows for early intervention. This proactive approach empowers doctors to implement preventive measures like lifestyle modifications or targeted medications before symptoms arise.

Personalized Treatment Strategies: Genetic testing results can inform treatment decisions. Knowing your specific genetic risk profile allows doctors to tailor treatment plans to maximize effectiveness and minimize side effects. For example, if a genetic test reveals you have a predisposition to high cholesterol that doesn't respond well to a specific medication class, alternative treatment options can be explored.

Risk Stratification: Genetic testing can help doctors categorize individuals into different risk groups. This allows for a more nuanced approach to preventive care. High-risk individuals can receive more aggressive treatment strategies, while those with a lower genetic risk may require fewer intensive interventions.

The Untold Truth: Limitations of Genetic Testing

While genetic testing offers valuable insights, it's important to understand its limitations:

Not a Crystal Ball: Genetic testing doesn't guarantee that you will develop heart disease. It simply reveals your predisposition based on your genetic makeup. Lifestyle factors, environmental exposures, and other genetic variations all play a role in disease development.

Incomplete Picture: Our understanding of the complex interplay between genes and heart disease is still evolving. New gene variants are continuously being discovered, and some genetic tests may not capture the full picture of your risk.

Psychological Implications: Learning about a genetic predisposition to heart disease can be emotionally challenging. Genetic counseling is crucial to ensure patients understand the limitations of the test and receive emotional support throughout the process.

A Case Study: Navigating the Nuances of Genetic Testing

Imagine Anabel, a 40-year-old woman with no family history of heart disease. However, she experiences persistent anxiety about her heart health. Genetic testing reveals a variant associated with an increased risk of heart disease. While this information is concerning, Anabel's doctor emphasizes that lifestyle factors play a significant role. Together, they develop a personalized plan that includes dietary changes, a stress management program, and regular monitoring. Genetic testing, coupled with lifestyle modifications, empowers Anabel to take a proactive approach to safeguarding her heart health.

Beyond the Test: Empowering Yourself with Knowledge

Genetic testing is a powerful tool, but it's just one piece of the puzzle. Here's how you can empower yourself with knowledge to navigate the world of genetic testing and heart health:

Seek Professional Guidance: Discuss genetic testing with your doctor to assess if it's right for you. Genetic counseling can help you understand the benefits, limitations, and potential implications of testing.

Understand Your Family History: Gather information about your family's health history, particularly regarding heart disease. This can provide valuable context for your doctor.

Embrace a Healthy Lifestyle: Regardless of your genetic makeup, adopting a healthy lifestyle – including regular exercise, a balanced diet, and stress management – remains the cornerstone of heart health.

The Untold Truth: Knowledge is Power

Genetic testing is not a magic bullet, but it's a valuable tool that offers a glimpse into your unique genetic predisposition to heart disease. By understanding your genetic makeup, you can partner with your doctor to

implement personalized strategies that empower you to take charge of your heart health. Remember, knowledge is power. Embrace the insights gleaned from genetic testing, adopt a healthy lifestyle, and embark on a journey of proactive heart health management.

The Evolving Landscape: The Future of Genetic Testing in Heart Health

The field of genetic testing for heart disease is constantly evolving. Here's a glimpse into what the future holds:

More Comprehensive Testing: As our understanding of genetics expands, future tests may analyze a broader range of genes and variants, providing an even more detailed picture of your heart disease risk.

Focus on Modifiable Risk Factors: Future tests may not only identify genetic predispositions but also highlight modifiable risk factors influenced by your genes. This information can be used to tailor lifestyle interventions for maximum impact.

Pharmacogenetics: A personalized approach to medication is emerging, where genetic testing can guide the selection of medications most likely to be effective and have the fewest side effects for a particular patient.

The Untold Truth: You Are Not Alone

The prospect of genetic testing can be daunting. However, remember you're not alone on this journey. There's a wealth of resources available to support you:

Genetic Counselors: These healthcare professionals specialize in explaining the implications of genetic testing and providing emotional support throughout the process.

Support Groups: Connecting with others who have undergone genetic testing or are managing heart disease can offer valuable support and a sense of community.

Patient Advocacy Organizations: These organizations provide information, resources, and support to empower patients to navigate the complexities of heart health.

The Power of Proactive Management: Embracing a Heart-Healthy Lifestyle

While genetic testing offers valuable insights, it doesn't negate the importance of a healthy lifestyle. Here's how you can take charge of your heart health, regardless of your genetic makeup:

Maintain a Healthy Diet: Prioritize a balanced diet rich in fruits, vegetables, and whole grains. Limit saturated and unhealthy fats, added sugars, and processed foods.

Embrace Regular Exercise: Aim for at least 150 minutes of moderate-intensity exercise or 75 minutes of vigorous-intensity exercise per week. Regular physical activity strengthens your heart muscle, improves blood flow, and reduces your risk of heart disease.

Manage Stress: Chronic stress can negatively impact your heart health. Find healthy coping mechanisms like yoga, meditation, or spending time in nature to manage stress effectively.

Maintain a Healthy Weight: Obesity is a significant risk factor for heart disease. Aim for a healthy weight through a combination of diet and exercise.

Don't Smoke: Smoking is one of the leading causes of heart disease. If you smoke, quitting is the single most important step you can take to protect your heart health.

Regular Checkups: Schedule regular checkups with your doctor to monitor your blood pressure, cholesterol levels, and other important health markers.

The Untold Truth: Your Heart Health is a journey, not a Destination

Taking charge of your heart health is a lifelong journey. Embrace the knowledge gleaned from genetic testing, prioritize a healthy lifestyle, and partner with your doctor to create a personalized plan for optimal heart health. Remember, small changes over time can have a significant impact. Celebrate your victories, big and small, and focus on progress, not perfection. By taking a proactive approach, you can empower yourself to write a new story

– a story of resilience, informed decision-making, and a heart that beats strong for a lifetime.

10.2 Personalized Treatment Plans: Optimizing Your Heart Health Journey

Traditionally, heart disease treatment resembled a one-size-fits-all approach. Medications were prescribed based on broad categories of risk factors, overlooking the unique biological tapestry of each patient. However, a revolution is brewing in the realm of heart disease management – the emergence of personalized treatment plans. This subchapter dig into how these customized strategies are woven together, considering your individual risk factors, genetic makeup, and overall health to create a proactive approach to safeguarding your heart.

Beyond Averages: Unveiling the Heterogeneity of Heart Disease

Heart disease manifests in a multitude of ways, with varying causes and risk factors. High cholesterol and blood pressure remain significant contributors, but the story goes far beyond these traditional markers. A patient's genetic makeup, lifestyle habits, environmental exposures, and even their gut microbiome all play a role. This heterogeneity – the vast variability in how heart disease presents itself – highlights the limitations of a one-size-fits-all approach.

The Power of Personalization: A Multifaceted Approach

Personalized treatment plans for heart disease are not a singular intervention; they're a tapestry woven from multiple threads. Here's how doctors leverage a personalized approach:

Understanding Your Risk Profile: A comprehensive assessment is the first step. This includes analyzing your medical history, family history, lifestyle habits, and potentially, genetic testing results. By understanding your unique risk profile, doctors can tailor treatment strategies to address your specific needs.

Targeted Medications: Gone are the days of a generic approach to medication selection. Personalized treatment plans utilize medications based on your specific risk factors and genetic makeup. For example, if genetic testing reveals a predisposition to high cholesterol that doesn't respond well to a specific class of medication, alternative therapies can be explored.

Lifestyle Modifications: Personalized treatment plans go beyond medications. Lifestyle modifications are crucial for managing risk factors and enhancing heart health. This might involve dietary recommendations based on your individual needs, a tailored exercise program designed for your fitness level, and stress management strategies to address your specific triggers.

Let's explore how personalized treatment plans address specific risk factors:

High Cholesterol: Treatment goes beyond a one-size-fits-all statin. Doctors may consider your genetic predisposition to cholesterol levels and prescribe specific medications, recommend dietary changes to lower LDL (bad) cholesterol and increase HDL (good) cholesterol, or even explore advanced therapies like apheresis for stubborn cases.

High Blood Pressure: Personalized plans go beyond a single blood pressure medication. Your doctor may prescribe medications based on your specific blood pressure profile, ethnicity, and response to different medications. Lifestyle modifications like weight management, dietary adjustments to reduce sodium intake, and stress management techniques are also woven into the treatment plan.

Inflammation: Chronic inflammation is a significant contributor to heart disease. Personalized plans may include anti-inflammatory medications, dietary modifications rich in antioxidants, and exercise programs to reduce inflammation and protect your heart health.

A Case Study: Tailoring the shade for Optimal Heart Health

Imagine John, a 55-year-old man with a family history of heart disease. He has slightly elevated cholesterol and high blood pressure. Through genetic testing, John discovers a variant associated with increased risk for heart disease. His doctor creates a personalized plan: a low-dose cholesterol medication, a tailored exercise program focusing on moderate-intensity cardio, and dietary modifications to manage blood pressure and promote heart health. This personalized approach addresses John's unique risk profile and empowers him to take charge of his heart health.

Beyond the Doctor's Office: Empowering Yourself with Knowledge

While personalized treatment plans are powerful tools, patient empowerment is crucial for long-term success. Here's how you can take an active role in your heart health journey:

Partner with Your Doctor: Open communication is key. Discuss your concerns, preferences, and any limitations you may have regarding lifestyle modifications or medications.

Educate Yourself: Learn about heart disease, risk factors, and treatment options. The more informed you are, the better equipped you are to participate in shared decision-making with your doctor.

Embrace a Healthy Lifestyle: Regardless of your treatment plan, a healthy lifestyle remains the cornerstone of heart health. Prioritize a balanced diet, regular exercise, and stress management to optimize your heart's well-being.

The Untold Truth: A Continuous Journey

Personalized treatment plans aren't static; they're a dynamic tapestry that evolves with you. As your health status changes, new risk factors emerge, or treatment responses are evaluated, your doctor can adjust the plan accordingly. Regular checkups are crucial for ongoing monitoring and refinement of your personalized strategy.

The Power of Collaboration

The journey towards optimal heart health is a collaborative effort, not a solitary pursuit. Here's how building a support system empowers you to navigate the complexities of personalized treatment plans:

Your doctor: Your doctor is your primary guide on this journey. Open communication and trust are essential. Don't hesitate to ask questions and voice your concerns.

Healthcare Team: Beyond your doctor, other healthcare professionals may be involved, like a cardiologist, nutritionist, or therapist. Working as a team ensures a comprehensive approach to managing your heart health.

Support Groups: Connecting with others who have similar experiences can be incredibly valuable. Support groups offer a safe space to share your challenges, celebrate victories, and learn from others on a similar path.

Family and Friends: Enlisting the support of loved ones can make a significant difference. Involve them in your healthy lifestyle modifications, encourage them to participate in activities that support your heart health, and build a network of support around you.

The Untold Truth: It's a Marathon, not a Sprint

There's no quick fix for a lifetime of heart health. The journey towards optimal heart health is a marathon, not a sprint. It requires dedication, consistency, and the ability to celebrate small victories along the way. Focus on progress, not perfection. Embrace the occasional setback as a learning opportunity and recommit to your personalized plan.

The Power of Proactive Management: Owning Your Heart Health

By embracing a personalized treatment plan, you're taking a proactive approach to safeguarding your heart. Here's how to empower yourself for long-term success:

Be Your Own Advocate: Become an informed advocate for your heart health. Learn about your risk factors, treatment options, and potential side effects. Don't hesitate to ask questions and be proactive in managing your health.

Celebrate Victories, Big and Small: Acknowledge your progress, no matter how small. Reaching exercise goals, making healthy dietary choices, or managing stress effectively are all victories worth celebrating.

Focus on Controllables: While some risk factors may be out of your control, like genetics, focus on the aspects you can influence. Prioritizing a healthy lifestyle, managing stress, and adhering to your treatment plan are all within your control.

Embrace a Growth Mindset: View challenges as opportunities for growth. If you experience setbacks or have difficulty adhering to your plan, don't give up. Reassess, recalibrate, and recommit to your personalized strategy.

The Untold Truth: You Are Not Alone

The journey towards optimal heart health can feel overwhelming at times. However, remember, you're not alone. By leveraging the power of personalized treatment plans, building a support system, and adopting a proactive approach, you can empower yourself to write a new story – a story of resilience, informed decision-making, and a heart that beats strong for a lifetime. Embrace the power of collaboration, celebrate your victories, and focus on progress, not perfection. With dedication and a commitment to a healthy lifestyle, you can rewrite the narrative of heart disease and embark on a journey towards a healthier, happier you.

CONCLUSON

"The heart is what makes life go. Without a heart, we would all be lumps." – Haruki Murakami

For too long, heart disease has been shrouded in misconceptions and a one-size-fits-all approach to treatment. This book has endeavored to unveil the untold truths about this complex condition, empowering you to navigate the landscape of heart health with knowledge and confidence.

We've sifted into the intricate workings of the heart, explored the diverse risk factors that contribute to heart disease, and shattered the myth of a preordained fate. The power to safeguard your heart health lies not in succumbing to fear, but in embracing a proactive approach.

This journey begins with understanding your unique risk profile. We've explored the power of genetic testing and the importance of creating personalized treatment plans tailored to your specific needs. By collaborating with your doctor and healthcare team, you can craft a strategy that addresses your individual risk factors and empowers you to take charge of your heart health.

This book is not merely a collection of information; it's a call to action. We've emphasized the power of a healthy lifestyle – a balanced diet, regular exercise, and stress management – as the cornerstone of heart health. Remember, small changes, consistently applied, can yield significant results.

The untold truth about heart disease is this: it's not an inevitable sentence, but a condition we can influence and manage. By embracing the knowledge within these pages, prioritizing a healthy lifestyle, and partnering with your healthcare team, you can rewrite the narrative of heart health. This book is your guide, but the power to write your own heart health story lies within you

Empower yourself with knowledge, embrace a proactive approach, and embark on a journey towards a vibrant, heart-healthy life. Remember, your heart is a remarkable organ, capable of immense resilience. With dedication and the right tools, you can ensure it beats strong for a lifetime.

REFERENCE

Chapter 1: The Untold Truth About Heart Disease

American Heart Association. (2023, November 17). Heart Disease. https://www.heart.org/

Centers for Disease Control and Prevention. (2021, February 25). Leading Causes of Death. https://www.cdc.gov/nchs/fastats/leading-causes-of-death.htm

Chapter 2: Unveiling the Complexities of the Heart

National Heart, Lung, and Blood Institute. (2021, December 1). Your Heart. https://www.nhlbi.nih.gov/

American Heart Association. (2023, August 31). How Your Heart Works. https://www.heart.org/

Chapter 3 & 4: Risk Factors Unveiled: A Multifaceted Approach

Mayo Clinic. (2023, May 12). Heart Disease. https://www.nhlbi.nih.gov/health/heart-healthy-living/risks

Centers for Disease Control and Prevention. (2022, March 31). High Blood Pressure. https://www.cdc.gov/high-blood-pressure/index.html

National Heart, Lung, and Blood Institute. (2022, September29).Cholesterol. https://www.nhlbi.nih.gov/health-topics/management-blood-cholesterol-in-adults

American Diabetes Association. (2023, June 27). Risk FactorsforType2Diabetes. https://www.niddk.nih.gov/health-information/professionals/clinical-tools-patient-management/diabetes/game-plan-preventing-type-2-diabetes/prediabetes-screening-how-why/risk-factors-diabetes

Chapter 5: Unveiling the Silent Threat: Inflammation and Heart Disease

Libby, P., Ridker, P. M., & Hansson, G. K. (2011). Inflammation and atherosclerosis. Circulation research,

107(8),1043-1051. https://pubmed.ncbi.nlm.nih.gov/35328769/

American Heart Association. (2023, May 17). Chronic Inflammation.https://www.heart.org/en/health-topics/consumer-healthcare/what-is-cardiovascular-disease/inflammation-and-heart-disease

Chapter 6 & 7: Sleep, Stress, and the Heart

American Heart Association. (2023, March 1). How Does Sleep Affect Your Heart Health? https://www.heart.org/en/health-topics/sleep-disorders/sleep-and-heart-health

American Psychological Association. (2020, August). How Stress Affects Your Heart. https://www.apaservices.org/practice/good-practice/stress-health.pdf

Mayo Clinic. (2023, April 12). Stress Management. https://www.webmd.com/balance/stress-management/stress-management

Chapter 8: Dietary Strategies for a Healthy Heart

American Heart Association. (2023, September 27). Dietary Approaches to Stop Hypertension (DASH) Eating Plan. https://www.heart.org/en/health-topics/high-blood-pressure/changes-you-can-make-to-manage-high-blood-pressure/managing-blood-pressure-with-a-heart-healthy-diet

American Heart Association. (2023, September 27). Mediterranean Diet. https://www.heart.org/en/healthy-living/healthy-eating/eat-smart/nutrition-basics/mediterranean-diet

Chapter 9: Exercise: The Heart's Best Friend

American Heart Association. (2023, March 1). How Does Physical Activity Improve Your Heart Health? https://www.nhlbi.nih.gov/health/heart/physical-activity/benefits

Centers for Disease Control and Prevention. (2023, June 6). Physical Activity Guidelines for Americans. https://www.cdc.gov/physical-activity-basics/guidelines/adults.html

Chapter 10: Precision Medicine: Tailoring Treatment to Your Unique Risk

National Human Genome Research Institute. (2022, April 27). Precision Medicine. https://www.genome.gov/

American College of Cardiology. (2023, January 24). Precision Medicine in Cardiology. https://www.ncbi.nlm.nih.gov/pmc/articles/PMC6021027/